MW01122821

Soar
Above it All

Overcoming Adversities in Life

By Sue London

Kristar Publishing
Burlington, Ontario, Canada

Kristar Publishing
2120 Salma Cres,
Burlington,Ontario, Canada
L7M3T1
1-888-812-1181
www.rockysjourney.com

Library and Archives Canada Cataloguing in Publications

London, Sue, 1962-
    Soar above it all : overcoming adversities in life / by Sue London ; edited by Judy Suke.

ISBN 0-9732158-2-8 (pbk.)

I. Suke, Judy, 1951- II. Title.

PS8573.O47Z467 2006   C813'.6   C2006-902506-1

Edited by Judy Suke
Cover design and book layout by Rod Schulhauser
Sue London's back cover photo by Axel Menzefricke
Printed by ISA (Interactive Solutions & Associates)

This book is dedicated to everyone who faces seemingly insurmountable challenges, illnesses, and a lack of faith. It is my hope, that through my story you will find your inner strength and the courage to soar above it all.

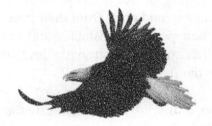

Testimonials

"I had the privilege of meeting Sue almost eight years ago. She came to me looking for a Fitness Trainer to help her gain the strength she needed to combat her fight against Crohn's Disease. It's amazing to see the journey Sue has taken over the years and see that she has done so with such a positive and fearless attitude.

When I read the title of Sue's book, "Soar Above It All", I couldn't help but start to understand the magnitude of her message. Everyone faces challenges in life, be it physical, mental, spiritual, societal, etc. It is what you do to triumph over these challenges that end up defining you as a person.

Through the telling of Sue's story, others faced with serious challenges can relate to and draw from their inner strengths helping them overcome their personal obstacles and grow as individuals. Sue has learned her true inner strengths and in this book passes them onto you as the reader.

Sue I'm so proud of you! You always saw the light at the end of the tunnel and have become an inspiration for so many others facing serious challenges. Never give up the fight, never stop telling your story and above all continue to grow as a shining light for others in need."

-Dave
Sue's friend and personal trainer

"Sue London has been involved in my spiritual journey, by sharing with me, her own spiritual journey. She has inspired to venture into uncharted areas of her soul and spirit. This book is an inspirational guide to the understanding of one's spiritual potential and their own personal soul's mission. I am sure that Sue's influential words and heart will inspire you the same way that it has inspired me. This book is a must to read!"

- Linda Powell
C.R., C.C.M.P.

"When I see the title, "Soar Above It All", I picture an eagle gliding high above the turmoil of the earth below. That is exactly what Sue's story is about. In this book, she bravely faces her past and all of its trials and tribulations and comes out of the darkness to soar above it all.

I sat beside her as she carefully chose the words that would bring inspiration to other women; to men; and to young girls. This is a story of the power we have within us to face all that life hands us.

I truly believe that by telling her own, painful story, Sue has shined a light that others may follow. Read her words, and you will know how to be strong; how to be brave; and how to overcome the obstacles, challenges, disappointments and disasters that you face.

In life, we will always struggle with both emotional and physical issues. Sue has lovingly, bravely, and spiritually written a story to help us … soar above it all. Read the book, share the story with others, and help Sue to spread her light."

-Judy Suke
Motivational Humorist
President of Triangle Seminars

Soar Above it All
-Overcoming Adversities in Life

Foreward

Preface

Acknowledgements

Chapter 1...	The Early Years	1
Chapter 2...	The Adversity Begins	6
Chapter 3...	Health Issues Appear	12
Chapter 4...	The Cycle of Life	14
Chapter 5...	Married Life	18
Chapter 6 ...	First House	21
Chapter 7...	Rocky Comes Home	24
Chapter 8...	A Desire for Children of My Own	26
Chapter 9...	A Death Sentence	31
Chapter 10...	More Help Is Needed	36
Chapter 11...	The Horrible Reality of the Disease	42
Chapter 12...	The Universe Brings Help	46
Chapter 13...	A Challenging Pregnancy	55
Chapter 14...	A Miracle Baby	61
Chapter 15...	The Marriage Breaks Down	65
Chapter 16...	The Car Accident	67
Chapter 17...	The Move	72
Chapter 18...	At Death's Door	77
Chapter 19...	In The Tunnel	83
Chapter 20...	A Different Me	86
Chapter 21...	Uncovering The Truth	89
Chapter 22...	Trying To Hold It Together	95
Chapter 23...	Taking Back My Power	99
Chapter 24...	Accepting Divorce	104
Chapter 25...	Jumping Through The Legal Hoops	106
Chapter 26...	Life Goes On	112
Chapter 27...	Not All Sunny Skies	117
Chapter 28...	Peace and Possibilities	120
Chapter 29...	Confident, Poised, and Powerful	124
Chapter 30...	My Earthly Angel	129
Chapter 31...	What if he is Mr. Right?	134
Chapter 32...	Goodbye Rocky	137
Chapter 33...	Combining Families is Not Easy	143
Chapter 34...	My New Career	146
Chapter 35...	Helping the Children Heal	148
Chapter 36...	The Beginning of Our New Life	153
Chapter 37...	Soaring	155

My final thoughts 161

A Collection of Quotes and Poems To Help You Soar 163

Recommended Reading 175

Foreword

I first met Sue London five years ago. At that time she was a single mom, recently divorced, recovering from a life-threatening disease, completing a Reflexology course, attempting to set up a new business, and striving to make sense of her past, present and future life.

One of her many positive characteristics, that struck me immediately was her positive mental attitude. After all she had been through, coupled with her then current circumstances, caused me to admire her determination to get on with life. Her journey during the past five years has been inspirational.

Sue has unselfishly dedicated countless hours helping people of all ages. She shares and teaches the importance of having a 'positive attitude'. She assists others in overcoming life's road blocks, while igniting their 'power of inner strength'.

Sue is an accomplished author, public speaker, active volunteer and supportive, caring wife and mother. She has written many articles for magazines and journals; published two children's books; appeared on television and radio; spoken to groups of all age, and raised money for various charities.

Sue London's book, "Soar Above It All," is her life story. It is a story of triumph over illness, abuse, disease and divorce. The book will help people move forward in their lives, heal, and become successful survivors of life's many challenges. Enjoy reading Sue's book and "Soar Above It All".

-Lloyd Oliver
Psychic and Life Coach

Preface

This book is not intended to inform you about what drug to take. It is not a medical book. In sharing my personal story with you, it is my hope that it will inspire you to believe in yourself, become a survivor, heal, and take your power back.

I was faced with illness, emotional challenges, and a lack of faith. I now know that it is through the trials and tribulations, the disappointments and disasters, the illnesses and accidents that we grow as human beings. Everything happens for a reason. My journey gave me strength and courage, and renewed my faith. The difficult situations taught me to go within and listen to my Higher Self. I can honestly say that I now have a life of great abundance. I have reclaimed my health, happiness and true love. What more can I ask for?

Acknowledgements

This book would not have been completed if it were not for the help of some amazing people. They all appeared when I needed them the most. I am extremely grateful and blessed by them.

To my loving husband, my soul mate, my best friend, Ross London. Our relationship started when you were my mentor at Toastmasters and grew into tremendous love. We have faced many challenges together. You are my strength, my support, and one of the greatest gifts God has ever brought me. I am extremely grateful to have you in my life. Thank you for helping me help others. I love ya, handsome!

To my children and stepchildren, you have all taught me valuable lessons. Through the situations you have faced in your lives, you helped me learn what I needed to teach others. You reminded me of all the good days and bad days that we shared; stories that needed to be in this book. A special thank you to you, Marie; for your patience and for cleaning and cooking so that I could write this book.

To my extended family, your love, lessons and challenges have tested my strength, confidence, and gifts. Thank you for helping me to become who I am today. To Keith and Bernice, you have taught me the meaning of family. Thank you for welcoming me with open arms. I am proud to now be one of your gang.

To my Grandpa Buck, and Johnny, two important teachers in my life, who have now crossed-over. Thank you for coming into my dreams regularly and reminding me of the lessons you taught me. I feel your presence many days and many nights. I miss you both very much. You will always remain in my heart.

To Lloyd Oliver, you coached me, you encouraged me, and you made me accountable. Years ago, when you suggested I write this book, I simply laughed it off. That was a time I didn't believe in myself. Well my friend, once again, you can smile and say, "I told you so." Thank you for helping me through the difficult times and being there at all the joyous occasions. You have been a wonderful friend.

Lloyd - lroliver@cogeco.ca

To Linda Powell, thank you for walking into my life at the right time. Twice I started writing this book and found it too painful to relive the memories. By taking a few of your Integrated Healing Therapy sessions, the painful memories were removed, helping me to complete this project. Linda, by your words of encouragement and your ability to continuously make me accountable, you gave me just what I needed. I thank you for your love and friendship.

Linda - lindapowellreflex@hotmail.com

To Judy Suke, a wonderful friend, who has certainly come into my life for a reason. I met Judy a few years ago while attending a networking event. She came up to me and said, "I can help you." Judy saw qualities in me that I didn't know I had. When I shared my dream of publishing my life story, without hesitation, Judy said, "When do we start?" Judy is a talented manuscript developer. Being intuitive she read my feelings and helped me to put this all together. We shared tears and lots of laughs while writing. There is no question in my mind that this lady is truly an angel from above! I love you my friend.

Judy Suke - www.triangleseminars.com

To my author friends, Karen Zizzo and Elfreda Pretorius, you have both given me wonderful suggestions and encouragement over writing this book. You made me be accountable to you. Your constant support and love has helped me face fears and challenges and go on to soar. You showed me by example the importance of our stories getting out there. You two give the word 'friendship' a whole new meaning. You bring me up when I am down. You ground me when I become unfocused. I am grateful to have you both you in my life.

Karen Zizzo - www.enlightenpublishing.com
Elfreda Pretorius- www.energyprinciple.com

To one of the best mentors Ross and I could ever have, Rod Schulhauser. Rod, you believed in me and my story. Without your faith, support, and talent, this project would not have been completed. Rod, you saw my future and simply said without hesitation, "How can I help you?" We are blessed that you walked into our life and are there to help us help others. People like you make our world a better place. Thank you for being you!

To all the people I met while I was working on this book. You helped me remember past situations and experiences that needed to be included in my story. Thank you for sharing your life with me and allowing me to give you words of encouragement. You have all been in the right place at the right time.

Because they have impacted my life tremendously, given me strength and courage, unconditional love, and eased my pain, I thank Spot, Rocky, Molly, and Willy, my furry friends. Having them at my side at all hours of the day and night while I have written this book has been wonderful. Each one of them has brought meaning to my life.

I have a huge thank you to God, for bringing me the people, the angels, the lessons, and the experiences. I asked for your assistance in my healing and you brought me healthy living. I asked you questions and you always sent answers. I asked you to bring me the people who could help me help others and you sent me the best. I am grateful for it all. Thank you from the bottom of my heart.

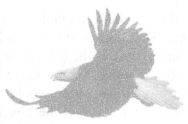

CHAPTER 1
The Early Years

"Some men see things as they are and say why. I dream things that never were and say why not."

-Robert Kennedy said at his brother's eulogy.

Growing up, I was an only child. I was extremely shy. I was always anxious whenever I had to be the center of attention. I remember actually feeling sick to my stomach simply because my kindergarten teacher was taking attendance. I would sit anxiously waiting in terror to reply, "Here."

As I got older I worried about everything. I worried about being late for school. I worried about being the last one to get my coat and boots off. At recess, I was afraid I would not hear the bell ring to come back into class. What if I didn't have time to eat my lunch? What if I didn't finish my work? What if I made a mistake? I was anxious, fearful, and had no self- confidence.

Fortunately, I had a pet. A dog I named Spot. She was a Terrier with white hair and had a huge brown spot right on her butt. I treated her like the sister I never had. I shared all my worries and fears with her. Spot knew all my secrets. She slept right on my pillow, under the blankets, and usually got more space in bed then me. That dog shed so much hair, that my mother kept the vacuum sitting close to the front door. She would vacuum guests before they left our house. Spot protected me from people she didn't get a good feeling about. She would growl and bite at people's ankles. Whenever she saw the boy next door, her hair stood on end; she would crouch down and prepare to attack. We never understood why until years later, when the boy confessed to me, that he had teased her whenever we would go out. While Spot was tied on a chain to our clothesline, he threw mud balls at her. I was not impressed!

When boys started coming around, Spot would let me know who was good and who was not welcome. She had great instincts. This dog had a mind of her own. She was actually a lot like me! I never got mad at her. We understood each other. We shared a strong bond and a love that will last a lifetime. For me, as an only child, getting a dog was the best decision my parents made.

Many people think that "only" children have it made. Obliviously they should get whatever they want and are spoiled. It really bothered me when people would constantly say how spoiled I was. That was not the case. I was disciplined and grounded many days in my childhood. Everyday of my childhood, I wished for a brother or a sister. It never happened. Spot was the closest I ever came. While on holidays, I never had a sibling to go with, or fight with in the back seat on those long car rides. This may sound funny to you, but, it was those types of things I longed for. I spent many days feeling lonely. Bringing an animal into your child's life can be one of the best things you can do for them. Trust me! Spot helped me to cope with those lonely days, gave me companionship, and built my confidence.

When we were looking for a pet, my mother wanted to get a dog that didn't shed hair. She called the local animal shelter, and decided we would get a poodle. The black curly hair Poodle bit me.

After that there was no way I wanted that dog! I was drawn to a skinny, lonely, sad looking Terrier. She sat all by herself, whimpering in the cage at the end of the room. Did she know what possible fate was coming the following day? Perhaps! When I walked toward her, she wagged her tail, as if to tell me to take her home. She had picked her new owner. At the age of three, I also knew she was the dog for me. I decided to call her Spot. When the man at the shelter told us that Spot would be put down the following day, if no one wanted her, I knew we were making the right decision. Poor Spot had been thrown out of a car window by the previous owner. She was scared and needed to be loved. I could do that.

I loved to be around animals. In addition to Spot I had fish, a turtle, and rabbits. I was literally compelled to rescue animals whenever they were hurt or lonely. When I was seven years old I was determined to make a positive difference for even more animals. My father helped me to prepare for a backyard children's fair. We had things to do, such as, a balloon dart toss, a fish pond, and a lucky spin board. Prior to the event, I went door to door in our neighborhood asking for any unwanted toys for prizes. I told everyone I could think of that I was going to have a fair with games for kids. They could bring their pennies and we would help save more animals. The fair was a huge success. This was the beginning of a burning passion that would last a life time. A passion to help animals and people in need.

To the world, my immediate family looked like a happy family. My mother was a 'stay-at-home Mom'. It was 'milk and cookies' after school, and homemade candied apples for Halloween. She sewed my clothes, knitted sweaters, and crocheted blankets. When Dad went out of town on business, we made it a family vacation. In public, they acted like a loving couple. I soon learned to play along and smile. In my heart, I knew it was a charade.

My parents were always there for others, while I struggled to get their attention. I would do things to gain their approval, and I would avoid doing things that were bad, to make sure that they were pleased with me.

My father was an angry person. I never knew when his temper would flare. Everyday when he came home from work, he was in a fowl mood. He brought his anger home from his job. He would complain, throughout our meal, about how many mistakes his employees had made that day. Our whole conversation during the meal was about him and his bad day at the foundry. I was always on guard as to what to say. My father scared me a lot. For no reason, he would fly off the handle and start getting angry, and then my mother would become silent and avoid him. If my father did something nice for me, I would hear about it for a very long time. He used those times to control me. If I said I didn't want to do something, he would remind me of all the good things he had done for me. I would feel guilty and then do what he wanted.

Dad was always working and never took time to enjoy life. He would literally create projects, and seemed to be avoiding time with my Mom and me. For the sake of clarity, I do want to acknowledge that despite the lack of closeness to my parents, they certainly assisted me in later years as best as they could whilst I struggled through physical and emotional challenges.

Throughout my whole childhood, next to Spot, I would have to say my best friend was my Grandfather Ross Hamilton, otherwise known as my Grandpa Buck. I called him "Bucky Baby!" He was so cool! He was my hero! I learned many positive lessons from him. One lesson he taught me was to have a system. He would always say, "Suzy, you always gotta have a system in life." At first when he told me this I didn't understand it, however, after hearing it repeatedly, I got the message. He was trying to tell me to get organized. Each day Grandpa Buck would come over for lunch, and bring another lesson with him. Growing up I hated to do math. I was not good at it, and felt it was a huge waste of time. This patient man worked with me until I got those addition and subtraction tables right. Then we went on to multiplication and division. He would teach me by using money. If I got the answer right, I got to keep the money! I think most kids would fall for this kind of learning!

Every Christmas, birthday, and when they returned from a holiday, my grandparents gave me a new doll. My favorite was a talking doll. You pulled her string and she would sing in French. Although, I didn't understand what she was saying, I thought she was so special. Grandpa Buck was one of the few people in my life I felt safe to talk openly with. I knew I could trust his advice. He always knew just what to say to put a smile on my face, make me feel secure, and let me know I was loved.

Another powerful man in my life was my Grandpa Smith. This was my father's Dad. Grandpa Smith was a man of honor, courage and strength. He had fought in WWII. He was one of the countless brave soldiers who fought the battle on the beaches of Normandy, France, in 1944. At a young age, I would listen to Grandpa Smith share his war stories and feel so proud of him. His military medals were representatives to the world, of his bravery and heroism. In my heart, he was already a hero and didn't need medals to prove it. After the war he suffered shell shock. It took him many years to heal from this illness but he did it. He was a survivor! I enjoyed visiting my grandparents' farm where I would run off into Grandpa's garden, sit and pick countless peas, and eat until my stomach was completely filled.

My Grandpa Smith died when I was only ten. In his final days, he would flirt with his nurses, and his mind was as sharp as a tack. His humor was a joy to listen to right up to the end. He died at the age of 92 and was buried on my Grandmother's birthday. He had taught me to have a strong determination, and had shown me that I should display courage in the face of every challenge that would come my way. If ever anyone showed courage it was certainly my Grandpa Smith!

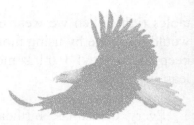

CHAPTER 2
The Adversity Begins

"Don't go through life, grow through life."

-Eric Butterworth

At the age of eleven, I was up at our cottage. My parents were cleaning up our property. We owned many acres of bush, with a cottage on it, and had to constantly pick up dead twigs to keep the property looking its best. One particular afternoon, my father insisted I help him with this clean up. I couldn't explain it, but, I felt tremendous fatigue in my body. It took all of my strength to walk across the room. When I told him I was very tired, and couldn't do it, he angrily said, "You are a very lazy kid." I don't think he knows to this day, how much that comment upset me. It made me feel he didn't believe me. Here my father thought I was being plain lazy, and I was truthfully feeling very ill. The overwhelming fatigue would come and go as the years passed, other symptoms would evolve, but I would not be diagnosed until I was twenty- six.

My Dad had a way of constantly belittling me, and putting me down. He would tell me I was fat, lazy, and would not amount to anything in life. My Dad had no idea the effect it was having on me. It is no wonder my self-esteem was low, and I had no confidence.

When I started grade six, boys began asking me out to the show and to go skating with them. A new boy at school, Jeff, who was half my height, and looked like a younger version of the singer, Andy Gibb, wanted to walk me home. I was not the least bit interested. The more he asked, the more I said, "No!" One day while walking home by myself, three girls from school ran up behind me, and started kicking me. They threw stones at me, and kept telling me to stay away from Jeff. I couldn't believe my eyes or ears. I was being beaten up, because of a boy liking me; a boy I didn't even like. This bullying from these three girls continued for a month. I told my mother about it. She said, "Walk home with a friend." I started out with a friend, but she took off when she saw the three coming. I was terrified to go to school. I was terrified to walk home. I had witnessed one of the three girls, Leslie, who was very tough, beat up another girl, after one of our baseball games the previous summer. She didn't stop at beating up girls; she even went after boys. The second girl, Kim, a real tomboy, took pleasure as she kicked me after she had knocked me to the ground. To this day, I have never seen such a mean look in someone's eyes. Kim's eyes were full of hate and anger. The third girl, Janet, a girl I thought was my friend, was the reason it was happening. I was shocked to see her turn on me. At first I had no idea why I was being bullied. Then I learned it was Janet, who had a crush on Jeff. She was jealous. No matter how many times I told her I didn't like him, she was still jealous. He liked me, and she felt I had to suffer as a result.

Unfortunately, I was full figured at an early age. Boys were attracted to my figure and it created problems. Many girls acted as Janet did. They wouldn't hang around me, because their boyfriends made comments of how good I looked, and they wished they were dating me. I had no desire to come between couples, however, the girls didn't want to believe it, and refused to take that chance. I never knew who I could walk to school with, hang around with, or have lunch with. Many times I would go by myself and sit in a quiet hall, eat my lunch, and read. This was my way of avoiding looking lonely. I felt very different from the other kids. Many kids were experimenting with drugs. That was something I had no desire to get into. I refused to be friends with the smokers. And the group that hung around the cafeteria, otherwise known as the "Jets," or snobs, was not a group for me. I certainly didn't fit in with the serious students, the group that always liked to study or was into science and math. I had a feeling I was going to do something important in my life, but just didn't know what it would be. I didn't want to do anything foolish that would affect my reputation later in life. When the other kids talked about their future careers, I would say I was going to get married and be around a lot of kids. I did a Career-Profiling test with my guidance counselor. The results specified that I should have a career in the health field, and had a natural skill for helping others.

When I was fourteen, Grandpa Buck convinced me to take my first part-time job working at a McDonald's restaurant. It was a wonderful learning experience that spanned two years. I learned many organizational skills and started coming out of my shell. I particularly enjoyed the employee activities. One of those trips included going on a dinner boat cruise around the Toronto harbor where I was able to create friendships with the other employees. Another benefit at McDonald's was the opportunity to work at various McDonald restaurants to experience their work habits and meet new people. In our training, we were told how important it was to be pleasant to the customers. I had no problem with this. I was a natural at this. I loved to talk with the customers and wish them a great day as I handed them their food with a smile.

While working at the McDonalds's restaurant I met my first love. A boy named Mark. I had been told by others there was a very cute boy, who thought I was very nice looking, and he wanted to meet me. Isn't that what every girl wants to hear? At first glance, I fell in love with this athletic, blue-eyed, adorable guy. Mark was the cutest boy in town. He had such amazing eyes, and looks that would stop you in your tracks. Before our first date I had him meet

Spot. He passed Spot's test! Spot thought he was the greatest. Mark had two Bull dogs himself. He certainly had a way with animals. We talked about our future, the children we would have, and growing old together.

Months into our 'perfect' relationship, one day at school, I noticed he looked strange. His eyes looked glazed over, he shuffled, and appeared numb to the world. That day, I learned Mark, the boy I thought was Mr. Right, was involved in drugs. I felt sick to my stomach. How could someone so smart, a person who wanted to become a lawyer, a person with the perfect looks, ruin his life with drugs? It was a terrible shock to me. Like my mother, I wanted to save the world, and my first mission was to save Mark! I stayed with him, and tried to convince him to get off drugs. It seemed the more I tried to convince him to stop, the deeper the addiction became. He would miss our lunch dates. Later I would see him falling over in the hall, higher then a kite, oblivious to me and the world around him.

I was angry at how Mark was wasting his life, but I never showed it. A part of me didn't want to lose him, and wanted to stick around to help him through it all. While, another part of me, wanted to run like hell to get away from all the bad stuff. I was sure I could save him. He never did the drugs around me. He knew I was adamantly against it. It seemed the more I tried to convince him to quit, the more he did it.

Mark picked me up for a hockey game one Friday night. After being seated for ten minutes, he got up and left without saying a word. He never returned to the game. About an hour later, I was given a message. An older girl, who knew both Mark and I, had called the arena to say, I needed to come quick. Something had happened to Mark. A friend drove me to where Mark was sitting slumped in the back seat of his car in the hospital parking lot. He was acting very strange. His eyes were rolled back into his head. He was drooling from the corner of his mouth. I was scared. The girl told me to get him away from this area. She only had her beginner's license and said she wouldn't drive and I was going to have to do the driving. I was only fifteen. I made a very stupid move. I drove his car back to my parents' house. Thank God I never got caught, or that would end my future for driving. How stupid we can be when we are young and in love!

We got back to my parents. I was worried about Mark and unsure as to how to help him. I told my parents the whole story. My father dragged Mark onto our front lawn and let him finish vomiting before bringing him into the house. It seemed like Mark was out on the lawn for hours. I found it difficult to understand why people take drugs and go through this nasty, painful, horrible experience. My father put Mark into my bed with newspapers all around the floor. I slept in the basement. They were not angry at me, they were concerned for Mark. My mother phoned his mother and told her what had happened. His mother was heartbroken, extremely worried, and very embarrassed that Mark would put our family through this.

During the summer he worked on a farm. He was either working, or with me, and he was away from the people who had been doing the drugs with him. I was filled with hope.

Just before school went back in that fall, Mark had a party. I thought it would be fun. Boy was I wrong! There were only a handful of us not doing the drugs. I hated how stupid they were acting. Mark saw the party was getting out of hand, and told me I would be safe in his bedroom. He said when everyone was gone; he would come and get me. At this point I was very scared, and wanted to get as far away as possible. That was not an option as he lived in the country. Half an hour later I heard a knock on his door. I opened the door, thinking it was him. I was wrong. It was another boy, Pat. I had known him since public school. He was very high. He walked through the door, and said he had been looking for me. "Mark was crazy to leave you alone," he said. His tone and eyes scared me. He pushed his stocky body against mine, and began to tug at my clothes. My terrifying screams could be heard above the loud stereo. Mark came to my rescue just in time. Although, Mark saved me, I will never forget that feeling of sheer terror. I knew I was about to be raped. Not long after that I started going to Jujitsu classes to learn self-defense.

I only saw Mark alone from that time forward. Never again did I ever go to a party with him. When he was not on drugs, he was the perfect boyfriend. He was kind and caring. A great catch for any girl! Mark and I were together for ten months, until he went on a school trip to Hawaii. He came back with a new girlfriend, a girl that I had known since Kindergarten. I felt betrayed by both of them. It broke my heart.

While living under my parents' roof, for many years, I could feel the tension between them. My friends noticed the tension also, and asked why they stayed together. They would put me in the middle of their arguments trying to get me to side with them. My father would tell me, "One day I am going to get a girlfriend." I knew he was all talk though. Watching them and experiencing the tension, I wondered about relationships. Why weren't they affectionate towards each other? Did they love each other? Would I be able to find a loving person who would truly care for me? Living in that home, I felt insecure, and unsure about the future.

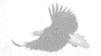

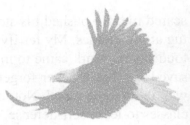

CHAPTER 3
Health Issues Appear

"Your children need your presence more than your presents."

-Jesse Jackson

My mother and I never had a good mother-daughter bond. I was unable to share my true feelings with her. As physical symptoms and health issues came up, she refused to accept them. Whenever I tried to have serious conversations with her, she would change the subject.

I was always low in iron and close to being anemic. In my late teens I started having bouts of constipation. I suffered tremendous, painful periods, accompanied with chronic diarrhea. Because I had no one to talk to, I thought this was natural. I learned later it was not. I started having debilitating pain in my joints. There were days when it was difficult to even walk. My doctor said it was because of growing too fast, and from being overly active in sports. I felt tremendous joy whenever I was playing baseball, swimming, or figure skating, and I certainly didn't want to give them up. I was quite a tomboy!

As I got older, I had no choice. I was forced to give up all sports activities to prevent the pain from getting worse. I could not even take part in gym class at school. Finally, coming to the end of grade twelve, when I was seventeen, I had to have surgery on my foot. The doctor had diagnosed me as having Freiburg's Disease. The bone had not developed properly in my foot. Due to severe pain in my foot; my walk was affecting my hips, posture, and my back. The procedure involved the removal of a bone in my middle toe, on my right foot. I was unable to walk for three months. When I was finally off crutches, I had to take physiotherapy in order to learn how to walk again. Not being able to walk for that period really opened my eyes. I realized how lucky I was to have two feet and legs.

Until a person has been on crutches, they don't realize how hard it is to hold books and open a door. It was difficult to walk down a crowded hall, trying to keep my balance, or go down a flight of stairs without dropping my books. Think about this the next time you see someone struggling with crutches. Give them a hand. I am sure they will appreciate it very much. I never took for granted the ability to walk ever again.

During my hospital stay I had a visitor. It was a boy from my English class. I was surprised to see Robert walk through my doorway; he was dating a girl I knew. During his visit he put down his girlfriend. I felt Robert was trying to tell me something. I felt he was coming on to me. Robert did share his interest in me. After I got out of the hospital, he told me he had broken up with his girlfriend. While home and recuperating from the surgery, Robert started coming over to visit me. He came over everyday after school. Spot despised this boy. She would growl at him as he walked up the driveway. She would bite at his ankles as he walked, and she would sit very close to me whenever he was around. She would protect me. At the time I didn't pick up on what she was trying to relay to me. I was going to make a mistake that was going to affect my future and Spot knew it! Our friendship grew, and we spent every possible minute together. Robert became my best friend.

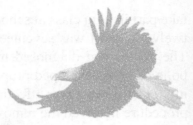

CHAPTER 4
The Cycle of Life

"To be upset about what you don't have is to waste what you do have."

-Ken Keyes Jr.

Four years later, on Valentine's Day, 1983, Robert proposed marriage. I thought it was about time. All our family kept asking me if he had popped the question yet. While out for a romantic Valentines' dinner I watched as Robert drank more and more wine. He was very nervous. This was unlike him to act this way. Finally just before dessert Robert took my hand and pulled out a ring and asked the question, "Will you marry me?" I replied, "Oh yah!" The next day the wedding date was set for June 16, 1984. An engagement party was thrown for us by our friends, George and Norma. I was given eight bridal showers. Life was very busy with all the planning.

Just four months before our wedding, Spot developed lumps on her belly. My mother told me they were nothing to worry about. "These lumps are just growths," she convinced me. The lumps got bigger and bigger. My mother's story never changed. Prior to Spot's death my mother was very quiet. She didn't make eye contact with me. I felt she was hiding something from me, but didn't know what it was. My mother made the decision on her own to take Spot and have her put to sleep. Apparently, Spot's belly was full of cancer for some time. Even at the age of 21, my mother felt I didn't need to know the truth.

I had secured part-time work for my mother, with me at the License Bureau during the busy months of February and March. After going to the Vet to put Spot to sleep, my mother came in to work and didn't make eye contact. She was even more quiet and withdrawn then the day before. Later that evening I understood why. I learned from Robert that she had taken Spot to the Vet to be put to sleep. My mother never gave me the chance to say goodbye to my dog, my best friend. Once Spot was gone, my mother never spoke of her ever again. I mourned that dog's death for a very long time. I would hear her bark. I would hear her paw scratching on the back door just after I had come in from outside. I had planned to have Spot walk down the aisle with me just months later when I got married. I felt a tremendous loss when Spot passed. I felt a piece of me was taken away. Spot was my friend, my support, and my strength. I had this dog come into my life for a reason. This dog helped me cope with a lonely childhood. She put a smile on my face when others couldn't. And now as I was preparing to walk down the aisle into marriage her role in my life was fulfilled. It took me many years to come to terms with what my mother had done. Not to be given the opportunity to say good bye to my best friend was a difficult thing to experience.

One week before Spot's death, Grandpa Buck's health started to deteriorate. He started talking about death. He said the day was coming when he would be reunited with his mother, who had passed away when he was only twelve years old. This kind of talk upset me. He told me, "Suzy, when I pass on, I will still be with you. I will be watching over you from above. I will always be there in your heart. I will live on in your memories. Keep my memory alive by sharing stories about me with your children." Without hesitation, I promised my future children would know him. Grandpa Buck scared me when he would talk like this. I never wanted to lose him. Grandpa Buck was my hero and heroes are not supposed to leave, or so I thought! Three days before his death he became bedridden. He felt tired all the time. He was having severe chest pain, but didn't want to go to the hospital. He was stubborn. When I called him, he would remind me of everything we had talked about and the promises I had made. I was 21 years old, stubborn, and confident I could pull him through this ordeal. I was in denial. I would phone him regularly. I thought if I could get him to come to the phone, he would feel comfort and strength from my voice. The night before Grandpa Buck died; I phoned to talk to my Grandpa. Grandma said, "Buck is in bed, and can't come to the phone. He is in great discomfort. There was nothing his doctor can do for him."

When I heard the phone ringing on that blustery early morning in February, I knew instantly something was terribly wrong. I heard my mother cry, "Grandpa Buck just died.' and my world collapsed. I felt dizzy, weak at the knees, and sick to my stomach. Within the span of a week, I had lost my two best friends, Spot, and my Grandpa Buck. I had no idea what to do, except to make egg salad for sandwiches. So, at 3:00 a.m., I started boiling eggs. My parents headed up to my grandparents, while I stayed at home with our neighbor, Mrs. Carroll. I didn't want to cry. I didn't want to feel the loss. I still wanted Grandpa Buck there at my side. I wanted him back with me.

I am sure Grandpa Buck saw his death coming, because in many of our last conversations he would always say, "Don't come to the cemetery and visit me. Remember me as I was when I was alive." I always got upset hearing this. I got mad at him for talking about it. I listened to my grandfather's advice, except for the funeral; I have only been at the grave site once. Grandpa Buck was right. He is not there. He lives in my heart. He lives through my memories and experiences. I see him in my children. I feel him around me in my daily activities. At his funeral the song, "Amazing Grace" was played. Every time I hear that song, I feel him with me. I feel him giving me a message to keep plugging away and to keep the faith. Throughout my life, I felt a stronger bond with Grandpa Buck then I did with my own parents. He died only four months before my wedding. I stayed angry at him for a very long time. I thought Grandpa Buck didn't care about my special day. I felt if it was important enough, he could have been there. He could have pushed his doctor to do more for him so he could get better. I know this was a selfish thought on my part. It was me grieving. It took me many years to come to terms with his death. I now accept that everyone and everything cannot live forever. He is kept alive through my words, feelings and actions. When Grandpa Buck looks down on me from above, I am sure he has a huge smile on his face giving me the thumbs up saying, "Suzy, you make me proud."

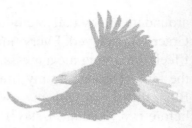

CHAPTER 5
Married Life

"Negativity only has power over you, if you allow it."

-Casey Combden

Although I was missing my Grandpa Buck, I was not nervous. I was sure I was doing the right thing. I was deeply in love with Robert. The 140 guests witnessed a typical wedding ceremony. We vowed to be faithful, in sickness and in health, 'til death do us part. We celebrated and danced the night away. Early the next morning, we flew to Florida for a week long honeymoon.

We began our new married life in a tiny apartment over a doctor's office. Our bathroom was so small; we had to open the vanity doors in order to sit on the toilet. You could not stand to take a shower due to the ceiling being on an angle. The apartment was cute; however, we rarely had company over due to the cramped space. I am telling you these details; because I watched other friends start out with a house. They would be strapped for money, with big mortgages. We didn't want to live like that. From day one, we decided to live on my husband's pay, and bank my pay for our first home, or any unexpected emergences. It was good we lived like this. It helped us to prepare for a future we sure didn't see coming!

A couple of months into our marriage, we started with a new dentist. All my life I had an older dentist, one that did no cleaning, and used all old techniques and tools. I was scared of this female dentist. She was not kind. As she cleaned my teeth for the first time she was yelling at me, telling me I should have taken better care of my teeth. I didn't know dentists cleaned teeth. I sure never saw my old dentist do that. By the time she had finished cleaning my teeth, there was blood all over the cloth bib around my neck, on my hands, and on my face. Seeing that sight almost made me faint! After she was finished, she told me I had three cavities. I was not impressed! This meant I had to go back to this horrible woman with the uncaring hands. Robert made the appointment. I had two weeks to prepare. My gums were raw from all the work she had done. I had to go home and avoiding chewing, I sucked my food. Two weeks came and went too quickly for my liking. She gave me three needles before she started the drilling. I was going through the roof with pain. I kept grunting at her to let her know that I was feeling it. The freezing had not taken. She refused to listen. I started to pass out in her chair. She got mad. She went out into the waiting room after filling one tooth and told Robert to take me home, never bring me back, and to find a new dentist. She refused to work on me ever again.

Robert yelled at me, all the way home. By this time the freezing had taken effect. I lost vision in my left eye, and could not hear out of my left ear. The search began to find a dentist that would take us. I wanted someone who was gentle and caring. I wanted to have a dentist that specialized in kids. I thought that would guarantee me this gentleness. We found a dentist and my other teeth got filled. Unfortunately for me, I was told I also needed my wisdom teeth out. I went home and cried. Another trip to the dentist!

The new dentist told both of us that we had to have some wisdom teeth removed. Robert had his removed first. His wisdom teeth were impacted. This made it a painful procedure for him. We

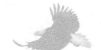

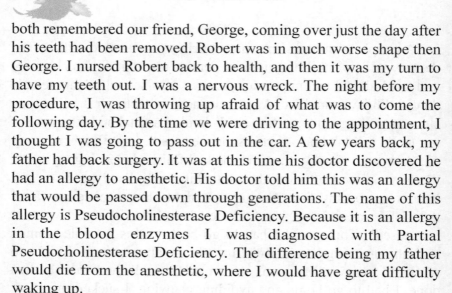

both remembered our friend, George, coming over just the day after his teeth had been removed. Robert was in much worse shape then George. I nursed Robert back to health, and then it was my turn to have my teeth out. I was a nervous wreck. The night before my procedure, I was throwing up afraid of what was to come the following day. By the time we were driving to the appointment, I thought I was going to pass out in the car. A few years back, my father had back surgery. It was at this time his doctor discovered he had an allergy to anesthetic. His doctor told him this was an allergy that would be passed down through generations. The name of this allergy is Pseudocholinesterase Deficiency. Because it is an allergy in the blood enzymes I was diagnosed with Partial Pseudocholinesterase Deficiency. The difference being my father would die from the anesthetic, where I would have great difficulty waking up.

Before my procedure started I reminded the nurse and dentist about this allergy. They told me all would be okay and for me to calm down. Easy for them to say! Even after me reminding them of this allergy, the nurse forgot to write it down, and it slipped the dentist's mind. This procedure started at 8:00 a.m. At 5:00 p.m., a nurse was walking me up and down the hall, trying to bring me back to life. The feeling I was experiencing was much like being in a fog, not hearing what people are saying to you, or seeing clearly through my eyes. It was a terrible feeling. Finally after the last patient was gone, the dentist felt it was okay for me to go home as well. I lost twelve pounds from the procedure. That experience made me fear dentists even more.

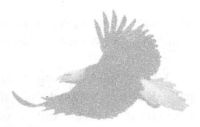

CHAPTER 6
First House

In 1987 we moved into our first house. It was a townhouse in a nice area. I was happy to be out of our apartment. We had a backyard. Robert and I enjoyed fixing it up and having friends over for parties. Our townhouse complex had a pool, so I was able to go out every evening for a swim. At the time, I was working at our local License Bureau. The job had both good days, and challenging days. Many people thought that I, personally, was the government and were angry at the rules they had to follow. My boss was a pleasant girl, but, she was a smoker. She always had a cigarette burning, and it often sat in an ashtray near. This made me feel tremendously sick each night. I had to put cold cloths on my eyes at night to stop the burning and the swelling. I found, as time passed, I had trouble breathing due to the second hand smoke. Because I was so against smoking, I was angry. How does one tell their boss they're not impressed? As more time passed, my breathing got worse, and I got angrier. I started having serious discussions with Robert about quitting. My health was much more

21

important to me than any money in the world. Robert feared that if I quit my job, we would have trouble making ends meet.

I lay in bed praying at night for a change to happen. I didn't have Robert's support, and that upset me. I had a difficult time understanding why my health was not important to him. Our thoughts were so opposite when it came down to things such as health and money. Deep down I felt if I stayed in this job, I could possibly end up with cancer due to all the secondhand smoke. My prayers were answered. One day, I was alone in the office. Two big, rough men walked in, and demanded that I transfer a vehicle into their name. I didn't get a good feeling about the whole situation. The ownership had not been signed off from the seller. I told them I was sorry and could not do the transaction for them. They became angry, and one man demanded, "If you don't do the transaction, I am going to use the gun in my pocket." My life flashed before my eyes. I thought, "No money in the world is worth this."

Thank God for the group of car dealers that just happened to walk in at the very moment. If it were not for them, I am not sure if I would have come out alive. The two scary men left and I stood there shaking uncontrollably. At this point, I didn't care if I had to live on the street. My life was very important to me.

When my boss came into the office, I told her about the situation. I then told her I was taking an early lunch. I never went back. I was too scared. My boss' mother took over working in my place. Years later my boss' mother died of cancer. Many believe it was from secondhand smoke! I prayed for resolution over this situation and God answered my prayers. Sometimes we ask for something and aren't prepared for what we get. I believe every situation teaches us a lesson. If we choose, we can grow from it and become a better person. Before the threat on my life, I didn't value myself. That situation opened my eyes. If you don't value and respect yourself, nobody else will. It was another lesson, I learned the hard way!

When I told Robert of the day's event, he was not happy that I had no intention of going back. He had a difficult time understanding why I quit. He told me I had to find another job. His lack of understanding and lack of compassion shocked me. I started questioning Robert's love for me. I thought, if it had been him in my shoes, I would have been devastated. Why were our thoughts so different? Why wasn't Robert devastated for me? Did this show a lack of love?

After being unemployed for a few months, and still trying to figure out what I wanted to do with my life, a phone call came from a girlfriend. Rhonda's maternity leave was ending and she needed to find a babysitter for her daughter, Terri. She asked if I would look after her daughter each day while she was at work. I thought it over, and decided to do it. Robert was happy I was finally bringing in some money.

My father was not happy with my decision. He felt the responsibility was too big. What if something happened to the baby? I was hurt by his lack of support.

It was a hard move for Rhonda to go back to work after Terri's birth. I wanted her to feel happy, not guilty, while at work. I told her how much I enjoyed looking after Terri. We were able to be out in the fresh air every day. I took Terri to parks and the library. This was the perfect job for me. I loved to be working with children. I then started doing home daycare through an agency in our town. I went through the process of having the Health Department check my home; a police inspection; and regular visits from the daycare agency. I was making more money than at the License Bureau.

I was looking after three little girls. Their ages ranged from six months old to three years old. I loved our time together. I would have to say I enjoyed being around children more than adults.

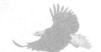

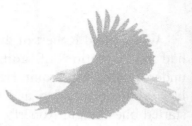

CHAPTER 7
Rocky Comes Home

"Those who bring sunshine into the lives of others cannot keep it from themselves."

-Sir James M. Barrie

The following January, a dear friend, Johnny Duncan, who was like a second Dad to me, came over and asked me to do him a favor. One of the pups from his dog's litter was returned from the previous owner. The owner worked in a mall and could no longer take it to work with her. She was going to have to put it to sleep. I remembered seeing the pup, and falling in love with it just after it was born. I hesitated. A part of me was still mourning Spot's death from three years earlier, and I didn't want to feel that pain again. Because of Robert's lack of love towards animals, he outright refused to let us take him.

Johnny was persistent, and assured me that by taking this pup, it would help me heal from the loss of Spot. This man had given me great advice all my life. I believed what he told me. My challenge was to convince Robert that it was the right move. It was not an easy task. Without hesitation, Robert again adamantly refused. Unlike me, Robert wasn't an animal lover. He didn't want any responsibility for a pet. And he certainly didn't like the idea of vet bills, dog hair, or dog dirt in the backyard to clean up. I was crushed when I heard his final answer, but refused to let it go.

Deep down inside me, I felt this dog was meant to be with me. I just knew there would be divine intervention in making it happen. After much discussion, and me agreeing to look after the dog completely, I won out. Johnny had given the dog the name, Rocky. I chose to keep the name.

When Johnny walked through our front door, it was love at first sight between Rocky and I. I immediately picked him up. He put his head on my shoulder, and placed his paws around my neck as if he was giving me a hug. He was dirty and badly in need of a bath and a haircut, but his eyes told it all. It was meant to be, for him to be with me, during this period of my life. At the time, I had no idea how much he would mean to me. After his first bath, Robert said Rocky would have to sleep in the kitchen. Rocky decided otherwise. He snuck up and slept on my pillow under the blankets just like Spot used to do. It touched my heart. It was the beginning of our strong, loving bond.

A few months after welcoming Rocky into our family, I began having terrible pain in my joints. Many mornings it was quite difficult to get out of bed. I was now babysitting four children. Ashleigh, our neighbor's four-year-old daughter was a new addition just months earlier. I thought perhaps I was getting too much exercise: fifty laps at the pool; playing on a baseball team; playing volleyball; plus sports and activities with the children I was babysitting. I was never one to sit still. I was also starting to have problems with hemorrhoids. This was something that I had never experienced before in my life.

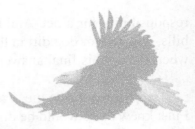

CHAPTER 8
A Desire for Children of My Own

"Never let the fear of striking out get in your way."

-George Herman 'Babe' Ruth

Babysitting all these children was wonderful, but I was longing for children of my own. I started talking about having children during our meals. Robert kept saying, "Not now, they are too expensive." Everything was money to him. It bothered me that Robert felt there should be no discussion around it. It was his way or no way.

Robert later changed his mind. Four years into our marriage, I became pregnant. I was thrilled. It was a dream come true. We had tried for approximately two years for this blessed event to happen. Because it was so difficult getting pregnant, I felt beyond thrilled when I got the phone call from the doctor's office saying the test results were positive! I will always remember getting that news. I was at a girlfriend's home, and had to sit down after the call and I cried tears of joy. It was the beginning of a perfect life. I finally would have it all! I knew I would be a great mother. I had gained much experience from looking after other people's children. I was going to teach my child positive values and help my child to become one of Canada's best citizens. I went home and told Robert of our great news. He was happy, but not as happy as me. I think a woman feels that miraculous joy in a more powerful way. Deep down I think Robert was seeing this situation as another costly venture. He would ask people with children how much this or that cost. A couple of days later, I received another phone call from the doctor telling me that there was a mistake. Someone had read the test wrong. I was now being told it was all a mistake. I sat down and cried. Just then, my mother walked in. She said everyone was wondering why I was not pregnant yet. Just what I wanted to hear! I learned later, I had miscarried. A month later I got a call from the doctor telling me this time I really was pregnant.

My bundle of joy would arrive in late March. I was ecstatic! Just in time for Easter. I felt I was being given the best gift from above! Weeks into the pregnancy I had the typical morning sickness, and chose to love every minute of it. I made the mistake of thinking I had to eat for two, and increased my eating intake. I ate double of what I used to. I drank a four liter jug of 2% milk per day. I craved cheese cake and ate it every chance I got. I couldn't get enough chocolate éclairs. I gained more weight than I should have. That caused me to develop more painful hemorrhoids. I couldn't sit on a chair without one of those blown up air cushions. Into the seventh month I started having difficulties. I started hemorrhaging. I also had a urinary tract infection. This baby wanted to come earlier than planned. My doctor ordered me to bed for complete rest for the remaining two months. I was also given antibiotics for the infection. I had to give up babysitting. It was hard for me to sit still and do nothing but rest. To sit and watch television all day, to me, was a complete waste of time in life. I remember lying watching the Olympics with my dog, Rocky, constantly at my side, giving me companionship and unconditional love. Because our house was a two story, I had to stay in my bedroom all day with the washroom on that level, and have my food supply for the day with me. As the weeks passed, my doctor allowed me to stay with my mother for the day. It was much easier as her house was on one level. My mother's neighbors, Mrs. Duncan, and Mrs. Carroll, would come over and visit me and help me pass the time. Mrs. Carroll, who lived across the street, was a lady I grew up knowing very well. Mrs. Carroll was like a second Mom to me. She and her husband were raising eight terrific kids. Boy, did she have patience and kindness. She would come over each day in the afternoon, and we would play cards. She would have all her dinner prepared in the morning so we could play cards longer. Mrs. Carroll made the best tea biscuits I had ever tasted, and every couple of days she would bring over a batch for us to enjoy. It was a much better way to put in the afternoon then watching television. Mrs. Duncan would share home remedies such as mint tea for settling my stomach, and hot honey and lemon for joint pain. She was the wife of Johnny. Mrs. Duncan was always a phone call away whenever Rocky was sick.

On March 27, 1988, I delivered a beautiful baby girl. I was in labor for sixteen hours. I had a difficult time in the delivery room. The baby was delivered with forceps. The more I pushed, the more she went back in. Robert couldn't handle the delivery and passed out on the delivery floor. Because of my allergy to anesthetic, my doctor could only give me gas for the pain. I have to tell you I sure loved that gas. I sucked back so much of it! During the delivery I ended up having 3rd degree tearing. My doctor had to call in a specialist to help repair the tear. My hemoglobin was very low. As a result I had to start taking iron supplements. I was anemic. After the delivery I was badly constipated. I had to have an enema. It sure wasn't pleasant, but it sure did the trick.

Lynn was such a blessing to me. When we brought her home from the hospital, I immediately put her on the floor for Rocky to check out. I didn't want Rocky to be jealous of the baby. He sniffed her and instantly became her guardian. He never left her side when she had her afternoon nap. Rocky let me know when she was awake and was in need of something. Rocky was becoming Lynn's Nanny.

I even enjoyed getting up for late night feedings. I loved quiet time with Lynn, watching her as our eyes connected. I felt an incredible bond. With Lynn cuddling into my body as she drank her bottle, I thanked God for giving me such a wonderful gift. I was unable to breast feed so this gave both Robert and I the opportunity to feed our new baby. It was such a happy time in my life. I found joy in everyday things. Watching Lynn as she slept, seeing her body stretch and wiggle as she woke up, and even observing her tiny face turn red as she filled her diaper, reminded me of miracles and put a smile on my face.

As time passed, I watched Robert spending more time alone with the baby, and less time with me. There was never an evening set aside to sit together, and have a conversation. Not that we really had ever sat and shared our day. Now, it felt like he had lost interest in me. It was something I couldn't explain, however, I definitely felt him withdrawing more each day.

We didn't have anyone to baby-sit, so going out on a romantic evening was out of the question. There simply wasn't money available for that. Every bit of his pay was accounted for; at least that is what he told me.

Rocky and I would take Lynn out each day for a nice long walk and enjoy the fresh air. I walked often, trying to lose the weight I had gained while eating for two. I was not having much success. In my naïve mind I thought that one loses all that weight within days of having a baby. Boy was I wrong!

Nine months after Lynn's birth I developed a lump on my eye lid. It grew bigger and more painful. It got to a point where I could not open my eye. I could not see out of that eye. My doctor referred me to a specialist. It turned out I had an allergy to smoke. My tear

29

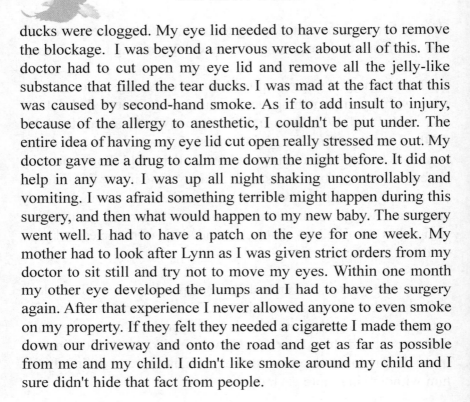

ducks were clogged. My eye lid needed to have surgery to remove the blockage. I was beyond a nervous wreck about all of this. The doctor had to cut open my eye lid and remove all the jelly-like substance that filled the tear ducks. I was mad at the fact that this was caused by second-hand smoke. As if to add insult to injury, because of the allergy to anesthetic, I couldn't be put under. The entire idea of having my eye lid cut open really stressed me out. My doctor gave me a drug to calm me down the night before. It did not help in any way. I was up all night shaking uncontrollably and vomiting. I was afraid something terrible might happen during this surgery, and then what would happen to my new baby. The surgery went well. I had to have a patch on the eye for one week. My mother had to look after Lynn as I was given strict orders from my doctor to sit still and try not to move my eyes. Within one month my other eye developed the lumps and I had to have the surgery again. After that experience I never allowed anyone to even smoke on my property. If they felt they needed a cigarette I made them go down our driveway and onto the road and get as far as possible from me and my child. I didn't like smoke around my child and I sure didn't hide that fact from people.

In January of 1989 I wanted to get serious and lose the unwanted weight. My doctor referred me to a dietitian at our local hospital. I don't believe in fad diets and wanted to lose the weight properly and in a healthy way. Within a month I started losing weight. I was very excited. My aunt, who also wanted to lose extra weight, started coming with me. We were supporting each other with our goal. We started noticing I was losing more weight than she was at each weigh-in. The dietitian was not happy about the rate at which I was losing. She told me it was not healthy for my body to lose so much so quickly. I had lost sixty pounds in less than three months. I began having diarrhea on a regular basis. As I kept losing weight, the dietitian and doctor became more concerned. I personally thought I had not looked this good since high school. During my yearly checkup, normal blood work gave an indication as to why I was losing weight.

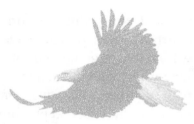

CHAPTER 9
A Death Sentence

I will always remember May 5, 1989. It was the day my life changed forever. I was diagnosed as having a chronic disease-Crohn's disease. I was 26 years old and married with a thirteen month old baby girl. When my family doctor said, "Your test results confirm you have a chronic disease," I thought it was the end of the world for me. She gave me the following meaning for this dreadful disease: "Crohn's disease is inflammation which penetrates the entire thickness of the bowel wall. It may attack at any point of the gastrointestinal system from the mouth to anus. Neither surgery nor drugs can cure Crohn's disease as it may recur in other parts of the digestive tract".

"Oh my God! I am going to die," was my first thought! There were tears in my eyes; my heart was pounding; I felt overwhelming panic. I felt dizzy and thought I was going to pass out right there in her office. I began to feel scared, very alone, and then angry at this rotten deal I was given. My mind started whirling with countless questions. How was I going to be a good mother to my baby? How

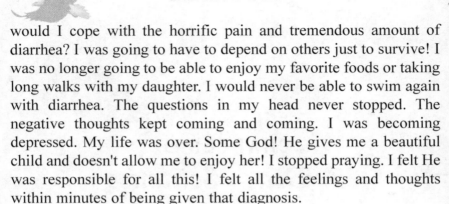

would I cope with the horrific pain and tremendous amount of diarrhea? I was going to have to depend on others just to survive! I was no longer going to be able to enjoy my favorite foods or taking long walks with my daughter. I would never be able to swim again with diarrhea. The questions in my head never stopped. The negative thoughts kept coming and coming. I was becoming depressed. My life was over. Some God! He gives me a beautiful child and doesn't allow me to enjoy her! I stopped praying. I felt He was responsible for all this! I felt all the feelings and thoughts within minutes of being given that diagnosis.

As I listened to my family doctor tell me my life was about to change, I began to feel more and more anxious, terrified and angry. I kept asking her, "Why is this happening to me? What did I do to bring this on?" My doctor could not answer these questions. I was her first patient ever to be diagnosed with this disease. Great I thought! I will be a guinea pig!

I knew this was very serious when my doctor asked me where Robert was. I could tell that she felt I was not taking the news too well. She was right. By the end of this first visit I was beginning to feel depression set into me. The question, "Why me?" kept creeping into my mind. I felt it was simply unfair for me to get this horrible illness at this time of my life.

I did some research. The symptoms of Crohn's disease is as follows: The most common is abdominal pain, which may be associated with loose stools and/or with decreased appetite and weight loss. However, some people may not have these problems. They may go to their doctor first because of unexplained fevers, sores around the anus, joint pain or swelling, poor growth or anemia. I did experience some of those symptoms.

The next day after the diagnoses I went out for a walk around the block. I found myself knocking on a close friend's door. Sandra and I knew each other as far back as our childhood. She knew about my doctor's appointment. When she opened the door she knew that something was terribly wrong by the look on my face. I thought it was strange that she would not let me come in. We stood in the doorway. She wanted to know what the doctor said. When I told her I was diagnosed as having Crohn's disease, she stepped into the house and began to close the door on me. She was only listening to the word, "DISEASE." Before I could say another word, she asked me to leave because she didn't want me to infect her or her one-year-old son. She didn't even give me a chance to tell her this was not a contagious disease. I was still in shock from the diagnoses and now feeling very confused and hurt by the reaction of a dear friend. Within 24 hours I lost my health, a good friend, and life changed forever.

Robert's family didn't comment much about my illness. My own parents were in shock, and wanted to know what caused it. My father called his brother, a doctor, to ask for details. My uncle was truthful about the facts regarding the disease. The frightening news shocked my parents. I think they also were hoping for less severe symptoms. Robert told me we would cope. I walked around in a fog for a long time after that.

Within weeks, I was rushed to the hospital with vomiting and severe diarrhea. I was dehydrated, and unable to keep food in. A nurse insisted she had the answer. She told me to eat lots of pudding. My instinct told me it was not the right thing to do, but she insisted, and actually forced it into my mouth. Within minutes, I had severe diarrhea. The bed was filled with it. Instead of the nurse being supportive, she yelled at me. She was angry that she now had to change the sheets, and help me get washed up. Just after that experience, I was started on a lactose-free diet by the hospital dietitian. I should have followed my intuition, and not taken the pudding. This taught me a good lesson… the answers are deep within us, but we don't always listen.

I later learned that not one of the nurses on that floor knew anything about Crohn's disease. In fact, some of them had never even heard of the disease. It was extremely frustrating for me having nurses look after me who were clueless. Some of them didn't understand how painful it was. This taught me to always ask the question, "What do you know about this?" or "What experience do you have with this."

During this time in the hospital, I was blessed to meet a very special nurse. She watched as I tensed my body every time I felt a wave of pain. My entire body tightened and I gripped the railing of the bed. She suggested that I try visualization. She explained that visualization is a technique, where one uses the imagination to cope with stress, take their focus off of pain, and activate the body's self-healing process.

She instructed me to think of a peaceful place that I had always wanted to visit. The place I picked was a beach in Hawaii. I had to use all of my senses to really feel this location. I had to smell it, taste it, hear it, feel it, and see it. I smelled the fragrant Plumeria flowers; I tasted the freshly-picked pineapples; I heard the waves crashing onto the shores; I felt the warm breeze brushing past my face; and saw the coconuts dropping to the ground.

Another visualization we used was to focus on a mountain scene. I was visualizing the beautiful Rocky Mountains in Vancouver, British Columbia, Canada. I would breathe in the clean, fresh air; see the snow covered mountain tops; pick the wild flowers growing on the mountain side; and feel the cool mountain air.

The more I practiced visualization the less pain I felt. Doing it took my focus off the pain. It took me away from it. If you feel sad, unhappy, or frightened, you can go to your favorite destination anytime.

The severe symptoms of Crohn's disease came on fast. My family doctor was surprised at the rate in which it was developing. She sent me to an Internist to assist her with my treatment. In the hospital, I was diagnosed as having a Perineal abscess after having a Gastro Intestinal Tract Series, otherwise known as a G.I. series. I did not enjoy these procedures at all. The tests involve Barium dye, which is shot into the intestinal tract through a hose. The dye reveals the abnormalities in the upper intestine on an x-ray. Because of the amount of diarrhea I was having, I found the tests extremely painful, not to mention very embarrassing. My dignity was taken away by Crohn's disease. It was the lower G.I. test that confirmed the inflammation was in the Ileum. The doctor ordered various drugs.

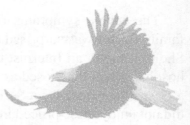

CHAPTER 10
More Help Is Needed

"Nothing can stop the man with the right mental attitude from achieving his goal; nothing on earth can help the man with the wrong mental attitude."

-W.W. Ziege

In June, my family doctor wanted me to see a Gastroenterologist. I couldn't understand why I was having to see an Internist, a family doctor, and now a Gastroenterologist, but thought my family doctor knew what she was doing. Having that many doctors made it very confusing for me. I was being told different things from each of them. It took up much of my time just visiting all of the doctors.

I felt an instant trust towards the Gastroenterologist. I was confident that he would be the doctor who would cure me. This was very important to me. Having a doctor that I felt comfortable with; someone who's judgment I trusted; someone who took the time to listen to my fears and feelings. We had a fabulous relationship. He allowed me to have a say in my treatments.

During my first visit he could tell I was in quite a petrified state. He sat me down and firmly said I needed to look at this disease just as part of my life. This was something I would learn to live with. He assured me I would be able to cope with it, and even have an active and happy life. He said I would learn to listen to my body, and eventually, I would know when I needed treatment, or increased medication, better than him. I was finding this hard to believe.

The doctor gave me a phone number to call, so that I could talk to someone who had the disease. Apparently, this person was supposed to be someone that gave support to others on a regular basis. He felt that talking to this person would ease my stress.

I was in denial. I thought I would wake up in the morning and this entire situation would be gone. When I got home I nervously dialed the number. I was afraid of what I might hear. Another part of me hoped that this person would tell me, "It is all a bad nightmare and nothing worse is going to happen to you." But I was wrong!

A woman answered the phone. I told her, I was just diagnosed with Crohn's disease, and I didn't know anything about it. I did not know how I was going to eat, or live, or be a good mother, with Crohn's. In the middle of asking different questions, the woman abruptly cut me off and bluntly said, "Realize this now! Having Crohn's disease is like having Cancer except you won't die from this disease. You will suffer in pain for the rest of your life." Wasn't that just what I needed to hear? Her words made me want to give up there and then. Words are so powerful. She totally depressed me. If that wasn't enough of a shock, she then told me she wasn't the one with the disease. It was her mother who suffered from it. Her mother had died six months earlier, and not even from the disease, but from natural causes. Can you imagine how badly this affected me? I hung up the phone and went into shock. What did I do to deserve this in my life? I cried continuously for two weeks. I went into a deeper depression. I wanted to give up. Let this be a lesson to you. Words are so powerful and can be so damaging to others. Always choose words of kindness to say to others.

At my next visit with the Gastroenterologist, he could tell I was in a worse state than before. He asked me what was wrong. I shared with him the details regarding the phone call. He was furious! He immediately had this woman's name removed from the support list. For six months she had been telling countless others the same line as she had given to me. Can you imagine how many people she affected in a negative way? My doctor was outraged. Once again he sat me down and said very clearly, "You can handle this disease! You are not going to die! This disease will become a part of your everyday life. You will be able to cope, and you will get through this. I guarantee it!" I had complete trust in this doctor and hung onto those words. "I guarantee it." My emotional state improved.

Over the next month, I made countless trips in the middle of the night, to the emergency department of our local hospital. I had to get shots of Demerol to help me cope with the intense pain, and Gravol to alleviate the vomiting. In 1989, many doctors and nurses didn't know much about the disease. Each trip to the Emergency Department meant different doctors ordering different blood tests. All of them kept telling me it was my appendix. It was extremely frustrating for me, knowing my problem, knowing what I needed, and having to wait so long to get it. I started feeling like I was becoming an expert in the medical field. I was using terms like 'dehydrated', 'blood count', and 'Upper G.I. Series'.

One doctor, who always seemed to be working in the Emergency Department during the midnight shift, had a really bad bedside manner. He had no clue about the disease and would always say, "Go home and sip water, and call your family doctor if it continues." I told him, that I knew I needed some blood work done, and I was dehydrated. After asking if I was a nurse, and getting the reply "No," he would always say, "When you become an

RN then you can make that request." Can you imagine how I felt having this situation be continuously repeated with this guy? Going to the hospital in the middle of the night meant phoning my parents, and getting them out of bed to come and stay with Lynn. Did this guy think I took pleasure in asking for help? I wish I had taken my power back, by taking control of the situation, and standing up to the doctor. Unfortunately, at the time, I didn't have the strength to do it. I learned from this that some doctors don't like patients to voice their thoughts.

The end of June I was admitted once again to the hospital. I had a fever, I was vomiting, and had diarrhea. I was anemic and had an abscess. I was treated with antibiotics and a sitz bath to help with the pain. I had been taking iron pills. The doctors now discovered that because of being anemic, the pills were causing the vomiting. I stopped taking the iron pills.

In July when I was back to see the Gastroenterologist, he put me on a drug called Prednisone, a powerful steroid. He could see the frustration in me and suggested Robert take our family on a mini vacation to get away from doctors, hospitals, and all those countless tests that I was put through regularly. Remember, I was seeing three different doctors all wanting various tests. When he first suggested this idea of a trip, I thought he was completely crazy, and had lost his mind. How could I travel in a car for any amount of time, when I couldn't even leave our washroom due to the tremendous amount of diarrhea and vomiting? He shared with me how many couples split up due to the stress of living with this disease. (One simply doesn't have any desire for intimacy due to all those unpleasant symptoms.) He told me that the Prednisone treats inflammation, and therefore, would help with pain and lesson the amount of diarrhea. I would have more energy, and more of an appetite. Although I experienced some bad side effects: excessive weight gain, round puffy face, some acne, mood swings and feeling restless, I can honestly tell you I feel that drug saved my life.

After a couple of days of being on Prednisone I felt a great improvement in my condition. I did have more energy. I didn't suffer as much diarrhea. I was able to eat food and actually keep it in. This was extremely exciting for me. I had so much energy, that I stayed up all night crocheting afghans for all my doctors. I could crochet a blanket in less than a week. It was a good way for me to have a positive focus and not feel frustrated that I was not sleeping. I was very happy with my doctor and completely trusted his advice. I decided that if he believed I could go on a holiday, then I would give it a try. Robert and I made arrangements and headed to Quebec City for a week's holiday. For my peace of mind, my family doctor gave me a doctor's name and hospital location in the Quebec area, and we purchased extra out of province insurance, just in case I needed it.

This seven hour drive did cause me to feel anxious and started my mind wondering those 'what if' thoughts again. I panicked every time I saw how far it would be to the next rest stop. "What if we didn't make it on time?" Anyone who travels on highways knows that a washroom is not always just seconds away. And with this disease, when you feel that cramping coming on, you know you need that washroom right now. We had to make many stops along the way. I thought if I stopped and used every washroom along the route, there would be less chance of an accident happening in the car. On the drive, I didn't eat or drink much. I wanted to keep 'empty', thinking that would prevent a quick trip to a washroom. This is a common feeling that people with this condition experience.

Our seven hour trip ended up taking approximately eleven hours until we got to our hotel. I felt tremendous relief to be at the hotel and near a washroom again. Even when I didn't need it, it was comforting to have it close by. On the third day of our trip I felt brave enough to go site seeing. We decided to go for a horse and buggy ride. It was a wonderful feeling, being outside again in the fresh, clean air, watching the leaves on the trees sway gently in the breeze. The temperature was comfortable with no humidity. (Humidity would cause me to have more diarrhea.) I enjoyed learning the history of the area, seeing the breath-taking sites, and trying to understand the language. I remember lying beside my baby, watching her have an afternoon nap. We were in a park, the 'Plains of Abraham', which was the site of a famous battle between the French and the English in 1759. We visited churches, ports, and museums in 'Old Quebec'. We even enjoyed a memorable lunch, at an outdoor café, while listening to musicians playing nearby. I had gone from, not leaving my bedroom and washroom, to enjoying life fully again.

I was grateful for having this experience, and for the doctor who had suggested it. This trip really made me start to see what was truly important in life. It is not the material things we have, but the little things that really count. It is taking the time to smell the fragrance of a flower, relish the sound of laughter, and see the joy on the face of a child. The memory of watching Lynn, having her nap in the 'Plains of Abraham', got me through many painful nights. I was grateful for being able to take this trip. It did prove to me that I still could have a life.

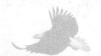

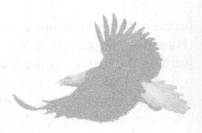

CHAPTER 11
The Horrible Reality of the Disease

"Most of the important things in the world have been accomplished by people who have kept on trying when there seemed to be no hope at all."

-Dale Carnegie

We were back from our wonderful trip one week when more problems started. I was nauseated all the time, having diarrhea again, terrible cramps, abdominal tenderness, hemorrhoids, and painful gas. I had also developed allergies and was having a constant draining sinus. I was taking a lot of drugs. When I first learned that I had Crohn's, I thought the diarrhea would be the worst symptom. I now felt that painful gas was much worse. I was extremely tired, not sleeping at night, and in constant pain. I was not able to go out, not walking or exercising, and just lying around. The gas kept building and building. When it came out, the smell was so strong and so awful, it even made my eyes water. I could clear a room. I mention this, because it was such an embarrassing part of the disease. It was difficult to deal with and I always tried to make light of it. I had no control over it. If I laughed, sneezed, or breathed heavily, or shifted in my seat, gas would come out. I would joke about it and blame my Dad, or my dog, Rocky. "That wasn't me, that was Dad." "How could you do that Rocky?"

The excruciating gas was worse at night. It was due to all the build up from the day of lack of movement. To help with the gas, I began drinking herbal Mint tea. It helped. Plus, I found it soothing on my stomach. When I experienced the horrendous pain, I curled up in a tight ball, and rocked back and forth on the bed. I cried out, begging Robert to do something. He felt helpless. There was nothing he could do.

Rocky was a great comfort. He instinctively licked an opposite area to where I had the pain. For example if I had pain in my stomach, Rocky would lick my face or my legs. This took my focus away from the pain. I then concentrated on the texture of his tongue, and its wet feeling on my skin. It was a relief having Rocky at my side all the time.

I could spend many hours at a time in our washroom. The diarrhea could last for two to three hours at a time. Just when I thought there was nothing left inside of me, the spasms would start again, and the diarrhea would continue. Because Lynn was so young I set up a play area in the washroom. Her toys would occupy her as I was being sick. This way I didn't constantly have to stick her in her playpen or her crib. Of course, Rocky would help me by keeping Lynn occupied. He licked her, and played with her toys. I was full of guilt for having Lynn see me like this, but, I had no other choice.

I was always full of guilt. My parents helped when they could. They gave up vacations and time with their friends to care for Lynn. I didn't want them to look after Lynn all the time. I wanted to be her mother, and look after her as much as possible. Lynn also spent a lot of time with our friend, Norma, and her daughter. I didn't feel as guilty when Lynn was with Norma for two reasons. Norma reminded me how easy it was for her when Lynn was over. Lynn would play with her daughter and this gave Norma a chance to get caught up with her chores. It was good for Lynn to be playing with another child, and doing normal activities.

The nights were the worst as I sat in the washroom hour after hour with chronic diarrhea and vomiting. It happened every night. I would sit on the washroom floor leaning over the toilet and wrenching into the toilet with Rocky at my side. Other nights I would sit on the toilet for hours having diarrhea while holding a bucket and vomiting into it. My dog pulled me through. His eyes would look deeply into mine and radiate love and kindness. I could feel his eyes telling me, we would get through the excruciating pain together. As long as he was there I knew I could cope.

The constant pain from this disease was getting harder and harder to handle. To give you an idea of how painful this disease is, if you have experienced labor and delivery, consider this one hundred times worse. Finding no solutions for the nonstop pain was really starting to affect me mentally. I was suicidal. I wasn't sure how to do it, but thought it would come to me. I didn't want my family to find me in a pool of blood, or hanging from a rafter. I thought that my family would be much better off without me. I felt I was causing them tremendous grief. I felt I was a burden to them. I did not feel I was a good example of a mother to my child. I could no longer take my daughter for walks or play in the park. Lynn would toddle into my room and put her tiny finger to her mouth and say "Shhhhhhhhhhhhh." She was learning from every adult who walked into our home that she had to be quiet because her Mommy was sick. That broke my heart. What memory would she hold of me in the future? The thoughts of suicide lasted about two months.

I was very anxious about going out, and being away from a washroom. It was like a phobia for me. It was tempting to avoid 'living'. I was cut off from the world, and different from others. I felt like a freak. I had no choice, I had to avoid certain foods and make special dietary demands. This made me feel conspicuous. It was hard on friends and family, and I always had to carry my own food. To add to my embarrassment, I was constantly rushing off to a washroom.

One evening Robert wanted me to go out with a group from his office. It was for dinner and bowling. At the time, I sure didn't have the energy to do any kind of sport, especially not bowling. I was not able to keep any food in. I would eat and immediately need to run to the washroom. I even ate many meals in the washroom. When I told Robert I was sorry, and was not up to it, his anger and frustration started to show. "This disease is ruining my life!" he shouted.

I got frustrated and had a difficult time understanding why Robert was not the supportive husband; he had been at the beginning. He was not the one suffering the pain in his body. He was not the one having chronic diarrhea. He was not bedridden and weak. Robert started to avoid being around me. He spent more hours at work. He went in early and came home late. He said he was needed at work on the weekends. When parties came up to do with work, Robert said it was for employees only. I later learned that was not the case, the other wives were there. I had a hard time understanding this behavior and was still just trying to survive. Robert's comments grew to be more and more spiteful. He often snapped at me.

When a person is deficient in minerals, vitamins and other sources this can affect you mentally. For me, I was anemic and had a B12 deficiency. Having a B12 deficiency made me scattered, and I had trouble remembering simple things. For example, one day I was driving and came to a red light. I was not sure if it meant to go, or stop. My doctor told me I had to be responsible and not drive when I felt like this.

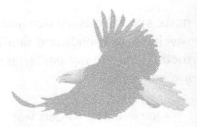

CHAPTER 12
The Universe Brings Help

"Failure will never overtake me if my determination to succeed is strong enough."

-Og Mandino

During my hours of frustration and pain, without even realizing it, I was constantly praying. "God, if you get me through the night, I will be a better person. I will be a good Mom. I will do whatever you want me to do. Please bring me help." Someone must have been listening. God, a spiritual guide, or a guardian angel answered my prayers. People started showing up in my life with lessons and answers to help me.

I received a coffee cup with words of encouragement on it.

DON'T QUIT

When things go wrong,
as they sometimes will,
When the road you're trudging
seems all uphill,
When the funds are low,

and the debts are high,
And you want to smile,
but you have to sigh,
When care is pressing you down a bit
rest if you must, but don't you quit.
Success is failure turned inside out,
the silver tint of the clouds of doubt.
And you never can tell how close you are,
it may be near when it seems afar,
So stick to the fight
when you're hardest hit
It's when things go wrong,
that you must not quit!
-Anonymous

Every cup of mint tea I had, I read this poem. It was a poem I read on a regular basis. It definitely helped me to keep going.

My Gastroenterologist was one of my greatest teachers. During one of my visits, he asked me to consider getting involved with a foundation that supports individuals with IBD (Irritable Bowel Disease). The name of the foundation is called the CCFC, (The Crohn's and Colitis Foundation of Canada). The doctor said by getting involved, I could get to know others with the same condition. He saw in me, a natural ability to relate to people and a generous spirit for helping people. He said I had 'a way' with people. He asked me to consider volunteering in different areas of the foundation. I was not sure what this 'way' was. Once again, he was right!

It was rewarding for me to be involved with the CCFC. I started giving support to others who were in need of some positive inspiration. In giving support to others, it helped me. I discovered that I did have a natural ability. Throughout the years, I have given support to over 2,500 people in need of encouragement or guidance.

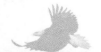

Through the CCFC, I was bringing awareness to the families of people with IBD. I honestly talked about the pain, the symptoms, and how to cope with the disease. Many people will not talk about this. They feel it is too embarrassing to talk about having chronic diarrhea. I was surprised to learn how many people suffered from IBD, or knew someone who suffered with it. It bothered me that it was such a 'hushed' disease. No one wanted to talk about it. There were so many unanswered questions. Many doctors did not even openly tell their patients, that they didn't have training in nutrition. Yet, they readily offered advice in that area. I was my family doctor's first patient diagnosed with Crohn's. She was honest with me and I was always sharing new information with her. This way she could help others in the future. Realizing these facts, I made a point of telling families what they would experience with this disease. Because they heard it from someone, who had experienced it, they accepted it. Many families thought their family member was faking symptoms. They were in denial and felt guilty.

I wanted to help find a cure. I took on the role of being President of a local chapter for the CCFC. To raise funds, I headed up the Annual Christmas Cake Sale. To help others learn more about how they could take control of their condition, and live life again, I planned educational sessions. Robert got involved with the local chapter also. We volunteered as a family, helping out at the Annual M&M's BBQ. We flipped burgers along side of the local politicians, and raised funds for the Foundation. It was also another way of making new friends. Spouses could share their frustration with other spouses. People, who were suffering from the disease, could talk to others, facing the same symptoms. We all learned that we were not alone. There were others with similar emotional issues. I found it was healing for me to do all this. It was taking the focus off my own pain, and my own troubles.

I learned to live one day at a time. When I got overtired, stressed out, upset or ate the wrong food, I did not have a great day.

I experienced pain, diarrhea, fatigue, and nausea. If however, I took care of myself, I had a good day. The choices I made created my day. This was a lesson for me. I normally put myself last. I didn't value myself. Now I had to rest when I needed to, and make the right meal choices for me. I could leave the dust and take a nap.

My guardian angel was working overtime one Christmas. I was taking sulfa drugs. I knew something was very wrong when I took the pills. I felt truly sick, and was vomiting. My family constantly told me to take them anyways. They said the doctor knew best. I kept taking them a few more days. The vomiting got worse. A voice inside me said, "Stop taking them." Because it was Christmas, it was hard to reach my doctor. I listened to the voice and stopped taking the drugs. My doctor later confirmed, that it was a good thing I stopped taking the drugs as they could have killed me. We discovered I was allergic to sulfa drugs. I would never take them again.

In 1990, I was ready to look for other options for healing. I was sick and tired of taking one drug to help ease the terrible side effects of another drug. I was sick and tired of being sick and tired. I knew there was more to life than always being sick.

The saying, "When the student is ready the teacher will appear", was true for me. At a family function, Robert's aunt, Cec, came up to me and said, "I do treatments that I think can help you." She was an alternative health practitioner. One of the methods she used was called, Reiki. She offered to give me treatments which would help me cope with the disease. I had nothing to lose, and lots to gain, so I took her up on her offer, and met with her. After our conversation, I started to feel hope that I could get off all of the medicine. I felt I had another option besides surgery and drugs with nasty side affects.

Robert drove me to the appointment. It took us a whole hour to get there. I sat in the passenger seat curled up in a ball, feeling like

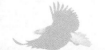

I was ready to pass out from the severe pain and cramping in my abdomen. I felt I was going to have diarrhea and vomiting at a second's notice. I was anticipating something horrible happening, if I could not make it to the washroom on time. I was focusing on the "what ifs".

I could not stand up straight, nor could I lay flat on my back. Cec had me lay on the table on my side with a pillow between my knees. I could handle this position. She put her hands on my head and had me take deep breathes. She encouraged me to breathe deeper, to go deep into my belly. This was something I had never done before in my life. I could feel stress leave my body with every breath I took. I was amazed. Within seconds, I felt a tingling travel throughout my body. My body became more relaxed and at ease. The pain and cramping grew to be less and less. I forgot about feeling anxious and about the "what ifs". It felt like I was floating on a cloud.

When the Crohn's disease flared up, I experienced many days where no food or liquid stayed in me after eating. After having Reiki treatments, I could eat and keep everything in. My mother would make delicious turkey dinners. I enjoyed them so much and now that I could keep them down, I could not eat enough. After so many months of suffering, it amazed me, how I could feel pain free, and have food stay with me. It was great to be able to eat and not have to run to the washroom. The Reiki treatments gave me hope. Reiki and Aunt Cec were truly blessings for me!

During my first visit, we talked for over an hour about my fears and worries. She helped me to realize how much emotional pain I held in my body. We talked about my childhood, Spot, and Grandpa Buck. I learned that thoughts directly affect our health. Fear and anger, towards my past, were literally creating my illness.

Reiki is pronounced "Ray-Key." Rei means "universal" and refers also to the spiritual dimension and the soul. Ki means the vital life force energy which flows through all that is alive. Reiki does not conflict with other health-care, but enhances its results. It does not interfere with traditional medical treatment, but facilitates benefits. Reiki speeds the healing process, and provides a source of restoring energy; while one is ill, under medical treatment, or in recovery. The best way to explain to you what happens is the practitioner places their hands on or over your body which allows the energy to flow through to the individual. The energy fills the Reiki practitioner's body first and then flows out through the practitioner's hands into the individual who is receiving the healing. A treatment is generally one hour in length.

Aunt Cec introduced me to two great books, "You Can Heal Your Life," by Louise L. Hay, and "Peace, Love, & Healing," by Bernie S. Siegel, M. D.

In Louise L. Hay's book, "You Can Heal Your Life," she says Colitis, (which is similar to Crohn's' disease), means insecurity. Problems in this area represent the ease of letting go of that which is over. I wasn't sure what I wasn't letting go of, but, I was very insecure. In the book, she indicated that chronic diseases represent the meaning of a refusal to change. Fear of the future. Not feeling safe. It was like she had read my mind. I feared the future. I feared the unknown! This book became like my bible. Whenever I had a pain, I looked up its meaning. There was always an affirmation to help me overcome the emotional issue creating the problem. For example, under Colitis, the affirmation is, "I am part of the perfect rhythm and flow of life. All is in Divine right order."

In Dr. Bernie Siegel's book, "Peace, Love, & Healing," it was confirmed to me once again, we can heal ourselves. Our minds do affect our health, and healing. Dr. Bernie Siegel, being a medical doctor, shared how patients can have power in their healing. He tells a story about a woman who wanted to have a meditation tape playing during her surgery. Although, the doctor fought against the tape being played in his operating room, the woman won out when

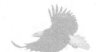

she stood her ground. She believed the tape would help her, and therefore it would. She had ever right to insist on having it played. Reading Bernie's book gave me strength. I felt a healing happen as I read it. I recommend this book to everyone!

Aunt Cec also suggested I get a juicer. She said by juicing my food I would get the nutrients my body was seriously deficient in, and I would start building my strength up again. Juicing vegetables was great for helping me keep my food in. Although, I turned orange from all the carrot juice I drank, it was an unbelievably, pleasant feeling to have something stay in my stomach. She also introduced me to a book called, "Food and the Gut Reaction - Intestinal Health Through Diet," by Elaine Gottshcall. Following this diet, I learned that keeping sugar out of my diet helped me to feel better. Below you will see 58 reasons why sugar ruins our health. I found these reasons opened my eyes, and not only convinced me to quit having sugar in my diet, but made it easy.

58 Reasons Why Sugar Ruins Our Health

1. Can suppress the immune system.
2. Can upset the minerals in the body.
3. Can cause hyperactivity, anxiety, difficulty concentrating and crankiness in children.
4. Produces a significant rise in Triglycerides.
5. Contributes to the reduction in defense against bacterial infection.
6. Can cause kidney damage.
7. Reduces high-density lipoproteins.
8. Leads to chromium deficiency.
9. Leads to cancer of the breast, ovaries, intestines, prostate and rectum.
10. Increases fasting levels of glucose and insulin.
11. Causes a copper deficiency.
12. Interferes with absorption of calcium and magnesium.
13. Weakens eyesight.
14. Raises the level of neurotransmitters called Serotonin.
15. Can cause hypoglycemia.
16. Can produce an acidic stomach.

17. Can raise adrenaline levels in children.
18. Malabsorption is frequent in patients with functional bowel disease.
19. Can cause aging.
20. Can lead to alcoholism.
21. Can cause tooth decay.
22. Contributes to obesity.
23. Increases the risk of Crohn's Disease and Ulcerative Colitis.
24. Can cause changes frequently found in people with gastric or duodenal ulcers.
25. Can cause asthma.
26. Can cause Candida albicans (yeast infections).
27. Can cause gallstones.
28. Can cause heart disease.
29. Can cause appendicitis.
30. Can cause multiple sclerosis.
31. Can cause hemorrhoids.
32. Can cause varicose veins.
33. Can elevate glucose and insulin responses in oral contraceptive users.
34. Can lead to periodontal disease.
35. Can contribute to osteoporosis.
36. Contributes to saliva acidity.
37. Can cause a decrease in insulin sensitivity.
38. Can decrease growth hormone.
39. Can increase cholesterol.
40. Can increase the systolic blood pressure.
41. Leads to decreased glucose intolerance.
42. Can cause drowsiness and decreased activity in children.
43. Can cause migraine headaches.
44. Can interfere with the absorption of protein.
45. Causes food allergies.
46. Can contribute to diabetes.
47. Can cause toxemia during pregnancy.
48. Can contribute to eczema in children.
49. Can cause cardiovascular disease.
50. Can impair the structure of DNA.
51. Can change the structure of protein.

52. Can make your skin age by changing the structure of collagen.
53. Can cause cataracts.
54. Can cause emphysema.
55. Can cause atherosclerosis.
56. Can promote an elevation of low-density lipoprotein (LDL).
57. Can cause free radicals in the bloodstream.
58. Lowers the enzymes ability to function.

Sugar Education
Quick Facts

◆Diabetes and other diseases grow significantly as sugar consumption increases

◆1900, average sugar consumption per person per year = 40 lbs

◆1980, average sugar consumption per person per year = 124 lbs

◆2000, average sugar consumption per person per year = 175 lbs

◆25% - 30% of our daily caloric intake is from sugar (empty calories)

◆More than 65% of our sugar intake is indirectly absorbed, i.e. beverages, preserves

◆A can of pop has 12 teaspoons of sugar

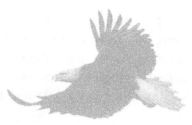

CHAPTER 13
A Challenging Pregnancy

"The future depends on what we do in the present."

-Mahatma Gandhi

With Crohn's disease, it is next to impossible to conceive. I think it is nature's way to protect our body. In January 1991, my health had improved, and the doctor told me the disease was in remission. My Gastroenterologist gave me the okay to try for another child. This was my chance. I stopped taking birth control. I was off the Crohn's medication. I was ecstatic. I never wanted Lynn to be an only child as I was. My excitement was short lived. In May I was still not pregnant. The allergies had gotten worse. I was now on a puffer every time I took Lynn to the park. I had developed a fistula and was now having recurring fissures. I was back on a multitude of medicines. The fistulas got worse and worse. I was referred to a surgeon. I was not impressed to say the least.

His diagnosis: I had three fistulas that needed to be removed as soon as possible. (A fistula is an abnormal passage from an internal organ to the body surface, or between two internal organs. Fistulas may occur in many sites from the mouth to the anus.)

The operation was scheduled for the following week. I was lying on the table. I remember the surgeon holding my hand. Soft, relaxing music was playing in the background. As I drifted into unconsciousness, I found myself feeling very peaceful. It was a feeling that I knew I would never forget.

Following the operation, when I came to, I looked down at my hand to see if the surgeon was still holding it. It felt like he was, but he wasn't. Was it my guardian angel? Perhaps it was my Grandpa Buck! Whatever or whoever it was, it sure gave me comfort and peace.

The surgery was done in my hometown. I was treated as an out-patient. After the surgery, I was home within approximately four hours. Three times, every day, V.O.N. nurses came to check on my condition, and change the dressings. Government health benefits also provided me with a homemaker to cook our meals, and clean. My mother had to look after Lynn, as that is something the homemaker would not do. We had no home life. Nothing was normal. The schedule for V.O.N. nurses controlled our days and evenings. They didn't consider how frustrating this was for us.

Within weeks, more fistulas developed. I was frustrated, having these nurses come into my home, disrupting any kind of normal home life. I was angry to hear the surgeon tell me, I had to go through more surgeries to remove the new fistulas.

On one particular day, a visit from a nurse changed my entire outlook. After reading my chart, she told me I was going to have to have another operation, and it would include a Colostomy. A Colostomy is opening the colon to the exterior and a bag is attached. I was absolutely horrified. I was 26 years old and I decided I had had enough with all these people telling me how my life would be run. I refused to believe this. She was insistent. In her opinion, I had no choice, and I had better face the fact she was right. She was pushy, arrogant, and rude. The ruder she got, the more determined I was to prove her wrong regarding me having that procedure. I was only a number to her. She didn't know me personally. What right did she have to diagnose my future? It had only been three weeks since the previous surgery. It was at this point, I truly saw how much determination I was born with. I made the decision I would fight this disease and win the battle against it. I started taking my power back. I started my journey towards healing.

Instead of having another surgery, I told the doctor I wanted to wait. I said I wasn't ready for it. I made this excuse up, to give me time to have more Reiki sessions. Aunt Cec and I put our hope and faith into the Reiki sessions. Instead of the normal one hour sessions, she would extent them to three or four hours at a time. Miraculously, the three fistulas healed. At a follow up appointment, with the surgeon, he looked at the x-rays and was confused. Immediately, he said, "There must be some kind of a mistake. The fistulas are gone!" I was sure he wouldn't believe my story of Reiki healing. I simply replied, "Really!"

In June 1992, my health had returned. I was off the medication once again. By the end of the month, I started feeling nauseated, was vomiting, and dehydrated. This time it was not the disease. I was pregnant! I think it shocked my doctors. My Gastroenterologist never thought he'd see this day. By the end of the month, I was admitted to the hospital, once again due to dehydration from chronic vomiting. Hormones play a role in this disease. When I was not pregnant, I was on birth control pills to control the hormones. Without taking them, my health would have been in worse shape. Periods would be irregular; I would suffer massive amounts of chronic diarrhea, and severe cramping. Now that I was pregnant, the hormones were acting up again. I was sent home for eight weeks and then admitted again. I was ten weeks pregnant, admitted for dehydration and weight loss. I was skin and bones. I had been vomiting on an average of seventeen times a day. I was extremely weak. I was treated with IV fluids and IV Gravol. It took thirteen days before I could keep any food or liquid down.

During this time I was missing my family, my normal life, and Rocky. I was getting more and more depressed each day. I was concerned about Lynn, being away from her for so long. I was sure this was hard on her, but I couldn't do anything about it. I had to focus on surviving and keeping the baby. The doctors asked me to consider the possibility of terminating the pregnancy, to save my own life. My weight was down to eighty pounds. Deep down in my heart, I knew I wanted this baby. My intuition told me that she was going to be a beautiful and healthy child. Without any doubt in my mind, I knew that I was going to live to enjoy her. I was determined Lynn would have a sibling. I kept telling myself I was pregnant for a reason. I strongly felt the pregnancy was part of God's plan for me. I had dreams of this special child, and two weeks into the pregnancy, I picked her name.

A family friend, Betty, from out of town, paid a surprise visit to me during this time. Betty and her husband were friends of my parents when they were kids. As I sat vomiting in my bucket in the hospital, she held my hand, and rubbed my back. She had tears flowing down her face. She said, "I feel helpless and wish I could do more for you. Life is not fair. You should not have to suffer like this." Although it was nice of her to visit and travel so far to see me, I felt depressed and exhausted after our visit. Because she was very negative, "the poor me" feelings came back. Instead of consoling me, she painted a picture that was even more dismal than the one I was seeing.

Because I was becoming more and more depressed, the doctors suggested that my family bring Rocky down to the hospital for a visit. At this point, I was barely able to get out of bed and walk to the washroom, just four feet away. Knowing Rocky was waiting on the patio down the hall, I refused to wait for a nurse to get me a wheelchair from another area of the hospital. Weakly, dragging my IV pole behind me, I inched my way down the hall, never letting go of the railing. I focused only on the patio door. As I got closer I saw my furry friend wagging his tail, jumping up on the glass door. I opened the door and he jumped into my arms. While we were cuddling, Rocky smothered me with kisses. My tears poured. It was at that moment, I knew I would be okay. My special friend, once again, had given me the strength to cope with a difficult situation. His unconditional love got me through. Although, I was still nauseated, I went home, and was able to keep food and liquids in. Rocky never left my side.

On March 23rd, Rocky was acting unusual. He kept pawing at his mouth. His teeth began to fall out. I thought this was very strange as he had just had his teeth cleaned a few days before. I took him back to the vet and learned Rocky had a broken jaw. The vet told me Lynn must have been playing too rough with Rocky, and as a result broke his jaw. I was horrified at this reason. Lynn was always gentle with Rocky. I told him he must be wrong. He stuck to his explanation. Rocky was kept over night to be observed. I went home and cried uncontrollably. It was obvious he was in a great deal of pain. I felt bad that Rocky was in such a terrible state. I hate to see any animal suffering. Knowing it was Rocky, just about killed me. A phone call from the vet, the next morning, got me even more upset. He told me I had to make a decision. I would have to pay $1500.00 for Rocky to have a surgery, where the vet would wire Rocky's jaw. If I couldn't come up with the money, my other option was to have Rocky put to sleep. I was not about to say good-bye to my furry friend just because he needed expensive surgery. I phoned Robert and told him the two choices. Without hesitation, with no concern for me or the dog, he said, "Put the dog to sleep." I strongly disagreed. He told me we didn't have the money to have this baby, where did I think the money would come from for the dog. I told Robert, "Rocky has been my savior, and I still need him!"

My mind drifted back to when I lost Spot. I was angry at myself for letting Rocky win my heart. I was pregnant, the hormones were raging, and I was sobbing uncontrollably. My mother returned with Lynn.

She took one look at me, and demanded, "What is going on?"

I told her the whole story. I explained the choices. I complained that Robert was not supporting me. My mother agreed that Rocky was good medicine for me. She felt that the issue with money should not end the dog's life. She left Lynn, and told me to enjoy the morning. She went directly to the animal hospital, and made arrangements to cover the cost of the surgery. Hours later, the vet called, and said the surgery was a success. Rocky was going to be okay. My tears began again, this time with relief. I was grateful for my mother's generosity, and thankful for the vet's kindness.

Rocky came home two days later and cuddled into me once again. He never left my side for days. He was different now. He wore a constant crooked smile due to the surgery. Years later, when the vet's assistant, was working at another clinic, she informed me that Rocky's jaw had been accidentally broken by the vet, during the teeth-cleaning procedure. I was upset, but there was nothing I could do then.

This entire ordeal was extremely stressful for me. I knew I had to be very careful not to let the disease get worse. The Prednisone was keeping things under control. I no longer suffered diarrhea, vomiting or nausea.

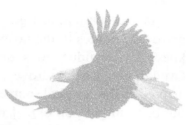

CHAPTER 14
A Miracle Baby

"Great hearts steadily send forth the secret forces that incessantly draw great events."

-Ralph Waldo Emerson

On March 28th, I had unexplained energy. I had not felt this energetic in years. I cleaned our house, made a delicious dinner, and went for a walk. Hours later, while watching TV, lying in bed, I felt a funny feeling in my stomach. The baby was kicking up a storm. I thought it was nothing. The C- Section was not scheduled until April 6th.

I felt a tightness and pressure in my lower back. As Robert focused on a "Star Trek" movie, I told him I thought the baby was coming. He snapped, "Not now, my movie is at a good point." Robert's movie was at a good point and my contractions were coming closer and closer. I started with the 'Hee's and 'Haa's. Rocky sat beside me licking my face as best as he could with his still tender jaw. I turned my focus to his licking.

As the contractions got closer, I started to panic. We had to drive 30 minutes to the hospital. There was a heavy snow storm. I knew if we didn't go soon, the baby could arrive in our car. Grudgingly, Robert drove me to the hospital. When we finally arrived at the hospital, nurses told me to hold my legs together or the baby might pop out. I remembered to tell the nurses that my Obstetrician had told me I was a high risk pregnancy. His orders were, when the time comes you will need a Cesarean Section. If I delivered naturally there was a greater chance of having a severe flare up of the Crohn's disease.

They quickly put me in a wheelchair and rushed to the labor area of the hospital. Robert was focused on finding a TV set with his movie on it. He didn't comfort me, do the 'HeeHee HaaHaa's with me, or support me. Although, he was right beside me, he seemed miles away. It felt like I was putting him out by taking him away from his movie. I wanted to say, "Don't bother coming into the delivery room, if it is just for show." Of course I didn't say that.

Before going into the operating room, the doctor gave me an Epidural. It kicked in right away. It took the pain away, and I told that doctor I was in love with him. If you were in labor and a doctor took your pain away, wouldn't you do the same?

Robert didn't hold my hand during the delivery, like he did with Lynn's birth. He couldn't see the surgery as it was shielded by a white sheet, however, he said that the noises bothered him. Robert was there in body during this labor and delivery, but not in spirit.

During the Cesarean Section operation, the doctor tied my tubes to prevent any future pregnancies. We had discussed this previously. Another pregnancy could kill me. I was not prepared to take that chance.

On March 29, 1993, at 12:02 am I delivered a beautiful baby girl, who I named, Marie. She weighed 6 pounds, 6 ounces, the same weight I was when I was born. I now had two wonderful daughters. I was exceedingly grateful for them. I felt truly blessed. I was overwhelmed with love. After Marie's birth, my Gastroenterologist paid a visit to my room. He had tears of joy in his eyes. We both felt this birth was a miracle. Because of me being so sick with this pregnancy, doctors gave Marie a thorough medical check over. I was terrified because of the amount of strong medications I had been taking during the pregnancy. I knew there was a possibility of complications. As the doctor stitched me up, I held my breath, waiting to hear news regarding my baby's health. The doctor, wearing a huge smile, brought me my beautiful daughter, and placed her in my arms. He told me she was perfect. I cried. I was relieved, grateful, and ecstatic.

Having had severe pain with Crohn's disease, made it easier to handle the recovery from the surgery. I bounced back to life the next day. I had never felt so good. Except for having stitches on my belly and a little discomfort, I was feeling great. Marie developed a bit of Jaundice after her birth but doctors were not concerned.

The day after Marie's birth, Robert brought Lynn into the hospital to meet her new sister. She had waited a long time for this day. It brought tears to my eyes, as I saw her instant love for her baby sister. There was an immediate bond between the two girls. This scene caused me to reflect over the past nine months, and all the sickness I had experienced. It was all worth while. I was able to give Lynn a sister, something I promised myself I would do many years earlier.

Marie and I were kept longer than usual to be monitored. We went home a week later. Because of the c-section, I was unable to lift heavy things for awhile. When I needed help from Robert, he would grunt and complain. He certainly didn't help willingly. He did not partake in Marie's baths, or feedings.

Robert worked longer and longer hours. He was distracted and distant. He didn't share in the same excitement that I felt over our new baby. The following November, when I broke my thumb playing volleyball he got mad. Robert was angry that once again, another excuse prevented me from fulfilling my regular duties. With a broken thumb, I learned how to change diapers with one hand and my teeth.

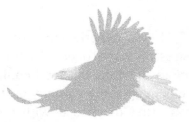

CHAPTER 15
The Marriage Breaks Down

"I can feel guilty about the past, apprehensive about the future, but only in the present can I act. The ability to be in the present moment is a major component of mental wellness."

-Abraham Maslow

Robert's anger began to upset me. What kind of a man was I married to? He was less and less caring each day. What bothered me the most was our lack of communication. We no longer had conversations. I wanted joy and happiness with plenty of love in our marriage. None of that was in it any longer. Robert never shared details of his day with me. Once again, he stopped taking me to company picnics and parties. He told me spouses were not allowed at the events. "The company is cutting back," he defensively said.

Later, I learned Robert had lied. I never put it all together. I was too busy focusing on the girls. Robert and I were living separate lives under the same roof. I never witnessed him bonding with Marie, like he once did with Lynn. I couldn't shake the feeling that something was terribly wrong. I just couldn't put my finger on the reason. I was too trusting and very naïve. I knew one day I would learn what was going on. It was just going to take awhile!

I was experiencing too much stress in my life. The biggest stressor was Robert. As time passed, it got worse. Robert grew more and more distant. I couldn't understand it. I thought it was me. Whenever there was any problem, I thought it must be me! When I was first diagnosed with Crohn's disease I found Robert to be supportive. He would go with me to the doctors appointments, hold me when I cried, and offer some support. He even helped me help others through the CCFC fundraisers. Slowly things changed. The more surgeries I needed, the more bad days than good days I had, and the more I couldn't do, the more he pulled away. When my diet created problems; what I couldn't eat versus what I had to eat, and how it had to be cooked (baked not fried), the more frustrated he became.   Robert resented the higher cost and blandness of this special diet. He found it hard to tolerate my need for constant rest. Because I was so absorbed in trying to survive, and be there for my children when I could, I didn't see how bad things were.

Eventually, after the birth of Marie, I lost lots of weight. I looked like death warmed over. I was skin and bones. My eyes were sunken in. My hair was falling out due to medication and the stress of the disease. I couldn't eat and I couldn't drink anything but sips of room temperature water at a time.

One depraved neighbor, who was always chasing after the women in the neighborhood, thought I looked like a model. One day he said, "You should be sick more often, because you look very sexy." Robert snapped back, "Looks aren't everything." Robert had lost all interest in me.

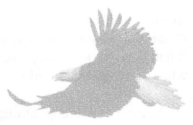

CHAPTER 16
The Car Accident

"Our greatest glory is not in never falling but in rising every time we fall."

-Confucius

When Marie was 2 ½ years old, she and I were out running errands. We were preparing to go away for a weekend to my parents' cottage. While making a left turn on a green light, things came to an abrupt stop. We were hit by a stolen car. The female driver was drunk, and on drugs. She came out of nowhere and hit my driver's door. I saw it coming and tightened my neck and left shoulder. This would cause problems later. After the woman hit us, she fled the scene. She did not even stop to see if my child was safe. A volunteer fireman, who happened to witness the entire event, came running up. He knew I was in shock, and kept me focused by asking me my name, what day it was, etc. The police officer, who was called to the scene, told me that I was one very lucky lady. He said if the other car had hit us two inches further back, I would have been killed.

The volunteer fireman took Marie and me to the hospital. I had damage to my neck, and was in shock. Once again I heard the words, "You are lucky to be alive." Marie was safe, healthy, and unharmed. Thank God! The doctor told me my body would feel like it had been hit by a Mac truck the next day, because I tightened up when I saw the car coming.

Later that evening, sitting at home, I reflected on the accident. I remembered that, just as the impact was about to happen, I saw two cloud like shapes, coming at me from above. At the time I found the memory confusing. I never thought much of it for a very long time until I saw a show on TV about miracles. The show talked about, how angels swoop down from above and save lives. There were illustrations of cloud like forms moving towards people. I know I did not put my foot on the brake. How did my car stop? At the time of the accident I thought the impact stopped the car, but I know I was wrong. She hit me on the side of the car. I stopped moving forward. Seeing the television show, made me flash back to that vision from the sky. Whatever, or whoever, came to my daughter's and my rescue, I am thankful. Am I a believer in angels after that? Oh Yah!

The day of the accident, when Robert was called at work, they could not find him. He never showed up at the hospital at all. I never learned where he was. The car had $3,000.00 damage and had to be towed away. I was traumatized, drugged, and unable to drive. It was a girl from his office that came to get us.

While Marie and Lynn played, I laid on our sofa in pain, and barely able to move. The doctor at the hospital had given me Tylenol #3's to take for pain. Robert got home hours later. He provided no explanation. When I shared the details of the accident, all Robert said was, "It was too bad you didn't get killed." I was in shock. How could he say such a horrible thing? I felt like he had stabbed me in the heart. His comment kept echoing in my head. I could not erase those painful words. How does one forget a painful comment like that? Robert never, ever apologized.

The Car Accident

When the doctor told me I would feel like I was hit by a Mac truck the next day, he wasn't kidding. I was black and blue from head to toe. Robert was no help. Our insurance coverage provided a housekeeper. She did household chores and cooked our dinner. She did not take care of the children. Thanks to friends driving me, I was able to get to physiotherapy.

I never shared Robert's hurtful comment, "It was too bad you didn't get killed." I was ashamed. I was hurt, and didn't know how to process it. I was afraid, if I told others how he spoke to me, they would tell me to leave him. I thought my parents would say I was a failure once again. I worried that they would say Robert wasn't good enough for me. Then, how would I cope, being alone, being a single parent. I buried this painful memory deep in my heart. Because I was emotionally abused, I felt alone, unloved, undeserving, ugly, and stupid.

Months later, the police contacted me in regards to the trial. I had to go to court as one of the witnesses against the woman who hit us. I arrived at the courthouse. My Dad came with me for support. A man walked up to me and introduced himself as the District Attorney. His eyes were kind. He made the entire process easier to deal with. I had never been in a courtroom before and had no idea what to expect. Remember I was a person who feared the unknown. The courtroom was filled with people. I sat with my stomach in knots. My case was the first one called. Lucky me! I had forgotten to ask the District Attorney where to go. My name was called as the first witness. When I got to the front of the room, I walked towards a box with a glass surrounding it and began to step inside. The judge wearing a huge smile, called me over to him, and suggested I sit beside him. Apparently, I was walking into the prisoner's box. Who knew! Certainly not me! Talk about feeling embarrassed.

The woman who caused this entire situation didn't show up for the trial. I was shocked. What nerve! The trial happened without

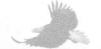

her. The judge questioned the police officer, who had been at the scene. He read his report. At the conclusion of the questioning, the judge handed down the sentence. The woman received a $640.00 fine. I was in shock. She had been charged with; stealing a vehicle; driving while drunk and on drugs; failing to stay at the scene of an accident; and did not appear for the trial. All of this was only worth $640.00 dollars. The District Attorney told me he had never seen a judge give such a steep fine. He thought the amount of the fine was higher, because the judge was appalled that the woman did not check the welfare of the small child.

I got home from that long day at the courthouse to find Marie had gotten creative with her hair. She had cut off all her beautiful, long, curly blonde hair on one side of her head. She stood in front of me looking so proud. All I could do was smile. She was alive and healthy, and that was all that truly mattered.

It took me four years before I could drive through that intersection again. Within a year the insurance company closed the file on the case.

Just after the accident, Marie started having dreams of Grandpa Buck. She would come in and tell me that she had seen him in her dreams. He was smiling at her. He never spoke to her, he just smiled. This was a man she had never met, yet, she vividly described him in every detail. She even described the colors in his favorite plaid shirt. Hearing Marie describe him sent shivers down my spine. I felt he was looking after her. He was her guardian angel.

I believe we all come into each other's lives for a reason. My second daughter, my miracle baby, was certainly a teacher to me. At the age of three she continuously told me, "Don't worry Mom." I never realized how much of a worrier I was, until she pointed it out to me. In all my conversations with people, I would say, "What if..." I would think of the worst case scenarios. Marie was wise beyond her years. She would tell me that worrying wasn't going to make a difference. She tried to get me to enjoy each moment. When we went for a morning walk, she stopped to smell every flower. At first it irritated me, and I told her to hurry up. "Stop dawdling, and let's go." The more I said that, the more she slowed down. I was certainly her 'work in progress'.

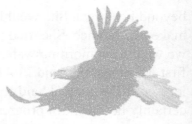

CHAPTER 17
The Move

"Whereversoever you go, go with all your heart."

-Confucius

Robert came home from work one day, and admitted that he only married me because he felt pressured. He said, because we had been going together for four years it was the only thing to do. It was either marry me, or break up.

I knew it was going to be another one of those stressful evenings. These evenings seemed to be happening every night. I wished I had listened to what Spot had tried to tell me, years before when she was biting Robert's ankles. She was telling me to get rid of him. After we were married, Robert told me how he hated animals. I should have seen the weakness in this man then and there, but I was blind to it all!

The next day, Robert came home from work, and told me he had decided we were moving to a new house. No discussion, he had made up his mind. I didn't question it. I was happy to get out of that townhouse. There was no privacy. The neighbors' children were running around, outside our front door, at all hours of the night and day. Children, younger then ours were out on their own. Children, ages two and three, left on their own to play on the street. I found it stressful always watching for cars. I grew more and more angry, trying to understand why the parents were not out there watching their children. The neighborhood was also becoming rundown. The only thing I would miss was the pool.

We sold our townhouse in three days. We bought our new house a week later. One thing I learned living with Crohn's disease is, don't leave anything to last minute. I never knew when the disease would flare up again, or I would have a run of sick days. Therefore, the day our townhouse sold, was the day I started packing up the house. It was Robert's idea to move, but I did all the packing and preparing for it. By the end of April, the house was completely packed. I forgot to leave out the kitchen supplies, so we ate many meals, at other family member's homes. Because I was organized, I didn't find the move stressful. Everything went smoothly, and I paced myself. I was determined to stay healthy.

June 21st, we moved into our new house. It was a side split, with a huge backyard, just a few blocks away. It was in a beautiful area, where everyone kept their properties looking their best. We had wonderful neighbors on both sides of us. It was such a positive change for us; I had high hopes that the move would improve our marriage.

A week after we moved in, the neighbor informed me that our house was bad luck. In every family that had lived there, the husband had an affair on his wife, and the marriages had ended in divorce. Not a good sign!

We had a lot of work to do on the house. It had not been loved in a long time. Five families had lived there. While doing landscaping and cutting back the overgrown bushes, we found skates and pop cans in the overgrown bushes. A broken down pool full of water had to be emptied, and taken down. The house was

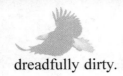
dreadfully dirty.

The upstairs washroom outside wall was rotted. Within a week of moving in, the entire wall had to be removed, and the rest of that room gutted. We then, could see into the garage below in some areas. We had to take showers with just a tarp protecting us from being in full view of the neighbors. It was a huge undertaking.

The living room stucco ceiling had been slashed with hockey sticks, and was badly in need of repair. There were three layers of wallpaper on all the bedroom walls, which took me many long hours to remove. I felt extremely tired in the evenings after doing the renovating all day. My side began causing me discomfort, but I tried to ignore it as much as possible. I enjoyed making the improvements, and didn't want to think about the 'what if' in my side.

I was working hard, and not getting enough sleep. The discomfort in my side turned to an odd feeling. After a lengthy week of removing dead shrubs and trees, I developed a tinge or pulled feeling. I went to see a doctor. He said, "It could be a torn muscle or something else." I didn't want to know what 'that something else' could be. This time there was no diarrhea but just severe pain. It almost felt like that of a baby's first kick. It didn't feel like it was Crohn's related, so, I continued working by covering my stomach with extra strength Tiger Balm to help with the pain. I kept my focus on the improvements on our home and not the pain that was increasing in my side. I kept telling myself that I had pulled a stomach muscle. Boy was I wrong! I was truly in denial. I didn't want to deal with illness and disease again. I didn't want to tell Robert of these unfamiliar feelings I was experiencing. I tried to hide the pain from the girls, but their intuition saw through it. They began helping me more with chores around the house.

Lynn read Marie her bedtime story as I spent time in the

washroom on the toilet. Whenever I shared difficulties with my health, Robert would become more distant and say, "What else is new." This move gave him a focus. He actually had conversations with me. It was always about simple things, such as paint color or floor tiles. However, I thought it was a start, at least some improvement in our marriage. Robert even wanted us to become intimate again. This was something that had not happened in over a year. I did not want to admit how bad the pain in my side was becoming, and made up another evasive excuse. My refusal increased the void between us, and it continued to grow. When I went to bed that night, I lay awake into the wee hours of the morning. I wondered what life would have been like for me, if I had married Mark, my first love. I knew it certainly would not have been this bad.

Coincidently, a week later, I ran into Mark, in a mall parking lot. I thought it was eerie how I had just thought about Mark, and there he was. As soon as we saw each other, we hugged. Time stopped as we stood there, holding each other tightly, while many memories flooded back. I was not thinking of the end of our relationship, but all the good times we had shared. He looked rough. He had extra weight around his middle. His hair was longer, and he wore one earring in his left ear. My first thought was, he looked like someone in a rock band. I, on the other hand, looked thin and many people thought I looked good like that. I hoped that Mark felt he had lost someone very special. He was in his late thirties, and had finally married a woman with two children. A part of me was glad that he had never had any children of his own. That had been a part of his dream with me. After catching up and searching for many answers in each others eyes, I finally asked the tough question, "Did you ever quit taking drugs?" To my horror, he told me he was still doing it. I exploded, "You idiot. When will you ever learn?" He got quite a lecture from me.

I was grateful. I was thinking, "What a mistake it would have been for me to have stayed with him. My life would have been

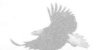

much different. Instead of being in a loveless marriage with emotional abuse, I might have had even less money, and a husband who sat on the sofa, doing drugs."

After my lecture, Mark gave me the apology I had been waiting many years for. He told me, "I spent countless days and nights thinking of the pain and hurt I caused you. You are the kindest person that ever walked into my life. I am very sorry for everything I did that caused you pain."

I appreciated the apology. It gave me closure, and allowed me to go forward in life. The lesson was hard for me to face. Not everyone is ready to heal and move forward. Some people like being where they are. Mark didn't want help. Years before, I had wasted valuable time. This was a tough lesson for someone who wanted to save the world!

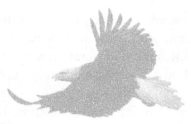

CHAPTER 18
At Death's Door

"Someday" may never come. So live each day better than the last. That way you'll wake up with so much excitement and anticipation you'll jump out of bed and shout. "I can't wait!"

-Bob Perks

The pain in my side grew more intense each day. Weeks later, I couldn't even roll over onto my side in bed. I was having tremendous difficulty breathing. I didn't want Robert to know how bad the pain was, because he would complain and withdraw. However, I knew I needed help. I didn't want to go to the hospital again, especially with how things were in our relationship, but I knew this time my health was in very bad shape. I could hear my inner voice, yelling at me to get to that hospital ASAP. The urgency I felt alarmed me. I convinced Robert to take me to the hospital where my specialist was.

It was a Sunday. The doctor was not available. I sat in the emergency department for three hours fading in and out of consciousness from the severe pain. I had a fever of 103 degrees. Finally, my name was called and they ran a whole series of tests. The tests results were not good. They said, the Crohn's disease had

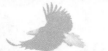
flared up, I had an abscess the size of a tennis ball between the 2nd and 3rd layers of muscle on my right side, and more seriously, my intestine had burst. Toxins and poisons were coursing through my body. I was immediately admitted.

Having studied spiritual beliefs, I felt responsible for my health. I argued that the Crohn's disease could not have flared up; the symptoms were not the same. Sitting there in the hospital I was angry for letting myself get sick again. I knew in my heart that this new crisis would ruin my marriage for sure. The doctor had explained how serious the situation was, and for the first time I was petrified. I realized that this time, I could die. The doctor prescribed a drug to calm my nerves and help me sleep.

Prior to surgery, they had to drain the abscess. During the procedure, a long needle is inserted through the stomach and into the abscess. The only way the doctor could tell if he had hit the abscess was by asking me to identify my pain level. Therefore, the procedure was done without pain killers. I am sure everyone in the hospital heard my screams as the needle hit the right spot. The pain was worse than when I delivered my babies. I was very angry at my doctor for putting me through that horrendous experience. I told him we were no longer friends. Although this procedure was necessary, I am sure he felt awful for causing the pain. After he did what he had to do, we were friends again.

Following more tests, the doctor came into my room, and told me the abscess was drained. The surgery was booked for the following day to have part of my intestine removed. I started thinking the worst. I was terrified. I thought about dying. What would happen to my children? Then I got angry with myself. I should have been able to control my emotions yet I had no control over anything.

In preparation to have the surgery, I had to drink four litres of a fowl-smelling liquid which tasted like baking soda. I gagged it down. The purpose of this unpleasant beverage was to clean my intestines out completely. I spent four hours on the toilet. During this time I felt nauseated, weak, and dizzy. I kept begging for them to let me die. A nurse and my father supported me and encouraged me to keep drinking. They had to help me off the toilet. My legs had gone numb from sitting so long. I was extremely weak and exhausted from such an intense clean out.

My father was teary-eyed. This situation was very difficult for him. Looking back, I am sure that he must have felt hopeless to help, fearful that I might die, and saddened by my suffering. This was a side of him that I had never seen before.

In order to comfort me and calm me down, the doctor told me, he treated my case and decisions regarding my health, as if he was making the decision for his own wife. He told me that he had found the surgeon who was most highly recommended for this procedure.

When the female surgeon walked into my room prior to the surgery I felt instantly comfortable with her. She reminded me of an angel. She had a calming and peaceful way about her. I asked her not to tell me what she was going to do. I didn't want to put any negative thoughts into my mind. I felt that when it was all over, they could tell me what they did during the surgery.

I asked my Gastroenterologist if he would go in, stay at my side and hold my hand, and not let me die. My fear was obvious. I begged him. He assured me I was going to make it, and reminded me that I had two very special kids and a dog at home who loved me. My nerves were completely shot at this point and I was doing a lot of crying. Robert was not there. I was alone. I was scared about so many "what ifs." I had told my doctor that I trusted his judgment completely. I just wanted his promise to let me come out alive, with no permanent bag attached at my side, and no blood transfusions. He promised I would live, but said he couldn't make any other promises. He couldn't control what would be needed during the operation. His assuring look and smile stopped my tears and comforted me.

During six hours of surgery, the surgeon removed three feet of my intestine and my appendix. I woke up with machines surrounding me, tubes in my nose, and a metal pole with a bag attached collecting my waste. To help me control the pain I was given "the morphine pump." The morphine was connected to an intravenous needle which was connected to a button. The morphine pump was to help me get instant relief when I started feeling pain. Instead of having to wait for a nurse to give me a needle, I could press the button and start feeling comfort much sooner. It did help with the pain, but it also gave me horrible feelings in my legs. It felt like bugs crawling under my skin. It made me hallucinate. I woke up one afternoon screaming after seeing countless snakes crawling all over my bed. Snakes, the one creature I dislike the most! It took a long time for the nurse to convince me I was hallucinating. It certainly felt very real at the time.

During my hospital stay, my father came to visit me the most. My mother came in less, because she was looking after my girls. I could see and feel how uncomfortable she was seeing me this way. I didn't want my girls to come in and visit. I didn't think it was good for them to see me hooked up to all kinds of machines. I knew the sight of me might traumatize them. It was very important to me, for them to have as normal a life as possible. I saw Robert twice over the eight weeks. When he would visit he kept his distance. He was not compassionate or supportive in any way.

As my health improved, I became more aware of my surroundings. The older lady in the next room was yelling constantly. I could not understand what she was saying, because she was speaking in a foreign language. She sounded fearful though. I asked the nurse what was wrong. I asked if I could help her in some way. The nurse told me the woman lived a life of sadness. She was a widow with children that never visited her. Her husband had died years earlier. Recently, she was diagnosed with Diabetes. Due to complications, she had just had her leg amputated. Because this older ailing woman didn't understand English, she didn't know exactly what was happening to her. She had no one to bring in her personal things such as a nightgown, toothbrush, or slippers. I could see why this woman was crying out.

I wanted to help her, but was not sure, what I could do, being in a weak state myself. I found it hard to believe that the hospital did not provide a toothbrush and toothpaste for this woman. The nurse told me it was the result of government cutbacks. It outraged me and I wrote a letter to our member of parliament making him aware of such an atrocity. No reply letter ever came. I decided my next visitor would be sent down to purchase a toothbrush and toothpaste for her. A week later, the woman was transferred to a nursing home to live out the rest of her lonely days.

I received a phone call from a mother of one of Lynn's friends at school. She said that she had overheard another mother loudly broadcasting how I lay close to death in a hospital. She said Lynn had overheard all of this. Where was this woman's brain? She didn't consider what her thoughtless gossip would do to my children! I was furious. I called my mother and asked her to have a talk with that mother and Lynn's teacher. My children were going through enough, without having to hear bad things from others. School was the one place where I thought they would have things normal or at least they should have. The woman's only comment back was, "Oh, I didn't realize Lynn overheard me!" If I had the strength, I would have ploughed that woman right in the face. I was very protective of my children and couldn't stand them being harmed in any way.

I found the days very long at the hospital. I missed my children, Rocky, and a normal life. I did not miss Robert. It was a relief to be away from him. I liked how I could escape his silence and lack of eye contact. Some days when I was not in as much pain, I visualized I was staying in a fancy hotel with room service. I would pretend I was in Hawaii. Thoughts like that helped me to stay sane. I had photos of my two girls and Rocky. The girls would draw pictures for me and send them down. I was anxious to get these pictures as I studied what they drew. I could tell by what they were drawing, how they were coping with my absence from home. If I saw happy faces, I knew they were doing well. If they colored with black crayon, I knew they were feeling down. We took turns phoning each other every night just before they hopped into bed. From somewhere deep inside, I would find the strength to put on my cheerful voice. I didn't want them to worry. Putting on a cheerful voice was the one thing I could do, to keep the disease from ruining their lives.

I missed having contact with other people I knew. I longed for some visitors. I did not have fragrant flowers sitting on my table, or many get well cards. I later learned, when people asked where I was, my mother told them I was away on a holiday. My friends and relatives had no idea what was happening. My cousin, Kevin, who was later diagnosed with Colitis, said he felt horrible that he was not there to support me. I really needed him, and he would have been there. He and I have always been so alike. We look like each other, act and think alike, and feel like brother and sister. He would have been the best medicine for me. I wish my mother had been honest with people. Perhaps in her own way, she felt that by living in denial, by not involving others, the situation would not be as bad. People cope with difficult situations in different ways. I personally needed support, love and encouragement.

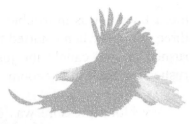

CHAPTER 19
In The Tunnel

"I find the great thing in this world is not so much where we stand, as in what direction we are moving. To reach the port of heaven, we must sail sometimes with the wind and sometimes against it, but we must sail, and not drift, nor lie at anchor."

-Oliver Wendell Holmes Jr.

About a week after the operation, when I started to feel some strength, I asked my nurse if I could take a shower. She got me a wheelchair and was ready to take me to the shower. However, I was feeling very strange, and tried to explain it to her. I felt dizzy, and unable to stay focused, and my heart was skipping beats. The nurse didn't want me to have a shower, feeling like that, and she made me rest for a bit before heading down. It had been a very long time since my last shower. I was really looking forward to it and did not want to let dizziness stop me. When the nurse returned, I told her I was feeling much better, which was not the truth. I was determined to have a shower. As we headed down the hall I began to feel worse. I thought it was best to let the nurse know how dizzy I was feeling. I didn't want to die in the shower, so I told her. She wrapped the cord of the call button around my arm while I sat in the wheelchair in the shower. The nurse told me to buzz if I started feeling any worse. Then she left. Although it felt terrific to feel water pour over me, I knew I was in trouble. I felt terrible. The nurse wasn't gone three minutes when I started feeling faint. I hit the button; the nurse rushed in, and caught me just as I was slipping to the floor. She rushed me back to my room.

My blood pressure was dropping drastically. I was no longer conscious. I felt I was drifting away to a place of peace and no pain. It was as if my body was no longer in the room. The screams of the nurses and doctors beside me, sounded like they were miles away. I couldn't hear the loud machines sitting beside me. For the first few minutes, I could feel someone pounding on my chest. Then I lost all feeling and saw a vision. The vision was something I had never seen before. It was a tunnel with a bright white light at the end of it. My body was floating. This magical place made me feel peaceful and pain free. As I was moving into the tunnel, a vision of my Grandpa Buck appeared. He was standing right in front of me, stopping me from going any further. It was wonderful to see Grandpa Buck again. My heart jumped for joy. I was confused. Why was he there? At first, I thought it was all a dream. With a look of intense concern, and yet enormous love, he told me I had to stop walking toward the light, and turn around and go back. He told me it was not my time to pass over. He told me I had great things to achieve in my life. I begged him to let me stay with him. He then spoke to me, "You have the final decision, but let me remind you of your two girls. How would life be for them without a mother, if you stayed with me?" Even in death, his words of wisdom helped me make the right decision. He had become my guardian angel. He promised he would always be at my side. I may not see him, but he would always be there. Once again, I trusted my Grandpa Buck, and followed his advice. Realizing my children would suffer, I decided to go back. The next thing I knew, I woke up in the hospital room. The nurses and doctors were shocked. They thought they had lost me.

I often wonder if I would have listened to anyone else, other than my Grandpa Buck. The angels knew what they were doing sending him. After all, in life, he was the only one I truly believed. He was the only one who was always honest with me. After my near-death experience, I really started thinking that there is an afterlife. I started to have faith, and feel that I was going to be looked after by a greater power, a power that I had stopped believing in years earlier. I was never the same again. I felt peaceful; knowing that I could overcome any adversity, set and achieve goals, and knew I had a mission to help others.

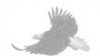

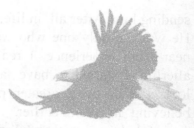

CHAPTER 20
A Different Me

"Knowing is not enough; we must apply. Willing is not enough; we must do."

-Johann Wolfgang von Goethe

On a rare visit, my mother-in-law and father-in-law showed me their true colors. I was heavily drugged. Before they came in, I was emotionally distraught. I wanted to go home. I was missing the girls terribly. I was crying a lot. I was begging the nurses to talk to my doctor and convince him to release me. I needed Rocky at my side, licking me and comforting me. In this state, a visit from the in-laws was the last thing I needed.

After my mother-in-law placed a bouquet of flowers on the table, she leaned over me, and all my wires and tubes, and whispered to her husband, "Well I would have to say Susan is not faking this. Perhaps she does have serious problems with her health."

What kind of a family was I involved with? I had a husband who didn't come to visit me, and a mother-in-law who didn't believe me. She later explained that for seven years she had thought I was faking the disease, in order to get attention.

I was furious! The new me was not going to accept this kind of treatment in the future. My life had been spared. I would focus on finding my purpose and not waste energy on people like this.

I came home in mid October. My neighbors, Betty and Earl, were doing their gardening, preparing for winter. Another neighbor, Les, was sitting in front of his garage drinking a beer. I didn't feel like I fit in with these people any more. I had been through an extraordinary experience, which was unlike any they had ever experienced. I was unsure what I would say to them. I felt disconnected.

My home did not seem familiar to me. It was like I was in someone else's house. I noticed how the girls had become more independent, keeping busy with their own activities, and helping out without having to be asked. I didn't know their routine anymore. I was familiar with the routine at the hospital and had come to depend on them. I was safe there. Now I was lost without the support. Rocky was the only one I was comfortable being around.

I was extremely weak, and still very helpless. My only support was my parents. My mother-in-law offered to help, but, I was stressed with her around, and didn't want her there. I couldn't shake the memory of her comment to her husband regarding me 'faking it'. I needed positive, fun people around me.

Things were worse between Robert and me. Because of my condition, my parents were always there to help. Robert resented their presence. He avoided conversation and refused to help me when they were gone. He put a wall up and completely closed himself off. On my first day home, I asked Robert for a blanket. My mother-in-law watched as he turned and walked away. She quietly said, "That is not very nice, Sue needs a blanket." Then she got it for me. His behavior shocked her, but she kept most of her feelings inside and only shared how I had caused many people much grief. She said to me, "This ordeal has been hard on him too, you know."

Unlike his behavior in earlier years, my father tried to keep conversations light and positive. I think he could tell I was having a difficult time being babied and treated me with kid gloves. My mother, stressed from looking after my children and trying to deny the true situation, she fussed around the house constantly cooking and baking. She did her best to cope.

The latest surgery had taken a tremendous amount of strength from me. By mid December, I was finally able to walk to the washroom which was right next to our bedroom. Slowly, I recovered physically. At Christmas, I was able to walk downstairs to our family room and watch the girls excitedly open their Christmas presents. Many Christmas' before the girls had to wait to open their stockings and gifts until I spent at least one hour in the washroom due to diarrhea. It didn't matter what time I got up, they were always waiting for me to open their gifts. This Christmas they didn't have to wait.

As the girls opened their gifts, I gratefully took in every sight, sound and smell. I watched Rocky crawl under the tree to get to his new stock of dog treats. I watched my mother and Robert in the kitchen preparing breakfast, while my father caught every moment on his video camera. I watched my Grandmother glance over her latest copy of the "Friendship Book." I thoroughly appreciated every moment and every detail. I was truly thankful to be alive.

By the afternoon, I was exhausted and had to lie down while the girls watched their newest Disney movie. I went to bed that night and thanked God for giving me the joy of seeing my girls open their gifts.

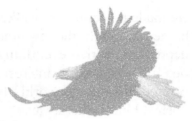

CHAPTER 21
Uncovering The Truth

"Defeat is not the worst of failures. Not to have tried is the true failure."

-George E. Woodberry

Strangely, the better my health got, the worse Robert treated me. He avoided all conversations with me. There was never any eye contact. He started doing things only out of duty and only when it was unavoidable. He was not paying our bills on time. He spent less time playing with our children. It was like my children were growing up without a father even though he was still living under the same roof. Robert lost focus and interest in our family's life. There was no more quality family time. Not thinking the obvious, I asked him to consider seeing our family doctor. I thought perhaps he had some kind of illness or was depressed. I knew the most recent stay in the hospital was difficult for everyone. I thought the stress of the latest surgery had gotten the better of him. The doctor put him on a drug that is used for depression. I learned of this two weeks later, when I found our youngest daughter playing with the medicine bottle he had left on the floor in a bag. I was angry with him over this stupid move and told him how irresponsible he was.

He made no comment, walked out the door, drove away, and came home late into the evening. Thinking he was suffering with depression, I tried everything to make him see all the positives in our life. He had no interest in this. Remember me, who always wanted to save the world? I thought I could help Robert. It only pushed him further away.

On September 6, 1997, I watched along with million others around the world as Princess Diana was laid to rest. I strongly related to her. We each held a secret of sadness in our loveless marriage. Like me, she had been married to a man who didn't love her, or even respect her. As hard as she tried to go forward in life, blocks kept occurring. Once, in an interview, I heard her say that she felt she was born for a reason. I could connect with that. I too had that same feeling of being born for a reason. I didn't know what my future would hold, but hoped it would not end in a tragic death like hers. This powerful woman gave me strength. I shed many tears as I listened to Elton John sing his farewell song, "Candle in the Wind." It was truly a touching moment for me. Princess Diana will be missed by millions, but forever loved by many. That's what I wanted in my life, unconditional love!

A week later, Robert announced that we needed to go to a marriage counselor. That was a huge shock to me. Sounds stupid I am sure. I was aware of the deteriorating state of our relationship, but never in my life had I ever expected to get counseling. I felt only others did that.

After going to the counselor, I saw no change in Robert or our life. When the counselor would ask Robert to make a commitment to do something with me, like going for walks, and making time for each other, he agreed in the office, but refused when we left. Robert told me everything cost money. He would continuously tell me money was something we did not have. I told him that doing something special for each other did not have to cost a cent. I would be thrilled if he picked a flower in our garden and gave it to me. I would be thrilled if he sat by the waterfront with me. I would be thrilled if he sat and told me about his day. The more ideas I came up with, the more closed Robert got. Nothing I said brought him back to me. He stopped wearing his wedding ring. When I asked him why he wasn't wearing it, he replied, "It is too tight." I didn't believe it. Robert had made the decision our marriage was over.

My neighbor, Betty, was very supportive during this time. I made excuses to her, telling her Robert had a rough time coping with my surgery and almost losing me. She was a retired nurse who had seen and lived through challenging times in her own life. She understood what illness can do to a family. Going through this was very difficult and extremely stressful. Although, we did not discuss all the details, it was nice to have someone to share a conversation with. I was ashamed to let people know, I was living in an unhappy home. I cried myself to sleep every night, while Robert stayed up watching television in the family room, until finally he fell asleep on the sofa. He would get up early enough, so that the girls would not see where he had slept. Robert thought he could cover up his lack of love, but children have a strong intuition. I am sure they knew their father didn't have loving feelings.

I didn't share my problems with anyone. I was too embarrassed. Friends, George and Norma, questioned why we were not getting together as much. Robert would make a lame excuse and brush them off. They knew nothing of our marital problems. They didn't even know we were seeing a marriage counselor. George was Robert's best friend; I didn't want to put them in a position to be choosing sides.

I knew if this stress level continued I would end up in the hospital again. I had to start looking at options for relieving the stress that was building up within me. I was never going to let myself have another flare up. Discovering that Robert's medical benefits plan covered massage therapy, I started having weekly massage therapy treatments to ease the stress.

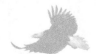

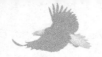

I had a great massage therapist named Mark. He was like a counselor to me. I found massage therapy to be very beneficial. I learned that massage has been used for thousands of years as a simple and effective method of attaining and maintaining good health, and its benefits have been recognized in many cultures throughout the world. The massage proved beneficial for my stress-related conditions, insomnia, and headaches. After I had my monthly B12 injections, I got a massage. I found by having a massage after my injection it helped me to feel the benefits of the shot much longer, and my energy level was higher longer.

After having these treatments I felt relaxed, stress-free and calm. I was very sleepy. I became so sleepy that I would struggle to carry on a conversation with my girls when I got home. This was the perfect medicine for me dealing with a bad marriage. After some treatments I would feel aches in my body. But by the next morning I was energized and ready to go. I had a bit of a headache after some treatments, but after drinking plenty of water this passed. Mark told me this was my body detoxifying, and it was a good sign.

I was able to share the truth with Mark. I told him about my pain and the terrible hurt in my marriage. I was ashamed to tell any friends or family, that Robert was treating me poorly. I was a failure. I had let people down by having this disease. I was not a good person. I felt ugly because Robert never took notice of me. All of these thoughts came from hearing those statements regularly come out of his mouth. "You are stupid... You are so naïve... I could do anything behind your back and you wouldn't know... I have no feelings for you... I have no life because of you..."

During the massages with Mark, it was a relief to get my anger, shame and hurt out. It helped to tell someone about the pain I was suffering.

It became a regular pattern, waking up feeling full of fear while covered in a cold sweat. I had terrible nightmares, reliving my intestine bursting, and other horrors, from the latest hospital stay. Many nights I woke up screaming after dreaming of being cut open. When I wasn't having that nightmare, then I was dreaming of Robert beating me and saying horrible things to me. I never shared these nightmares with anyone. I thought people would think I was crazy.

When I was alone and everyone was asleep, I made regular phone calls to the Local Woman's Shelter. I asked for my options. I had no money of my own. I didn't want to lose my home, leave my dog, or upset my children. One evening I saw a commercial on TV advertising how there is help available to those in need. Desperately, I called and spoke to the operator. She was with the Mormon Church and was offering free Bibles and other literature. She sent it; but it didn't give me the strength I was looking for. When she called me back a week later to make sure I had received it, I told her that I had, and unfortunately it hadn't helped and I explained my situation. She told me some things are not meant to be and to keep your faith. It was a very difficult time for me emotionally.

During a private session with the marriage counselor, he asked me a question which puzzled me. He asked me, "Why don't you see yourself as pretty?" I thought this guy needed his glass prescription checked. The counselor explained that when a person goes through emotional abuse, they are not able to see their positive traits. I tried to convince him I didn't have any. This concerned him. He told me to consider creating a new life. "There are many wonderful men in the world, and you sure don't have one of them." I was shocked by his words. He went on to say, "You are a very trusting but naïve soul. You have a lot of love to offer the right person."

I was confused at this point. I wasn't sure where he was going with all of these statements. He asked me to ask myself, what a husband would be doing for so many long hours at work. He asked me if I ever confirmed he was in the office. Finally by the end of the session, a light bulb went on. Robert was having an affair! I was in shock, just months before, I survived a near death experience, and now to learn this. It made sense why he was never around; why he was not making eye contact; and why he was disconnecting himself from the children and me. Other people had joy, love, and happiness in their life. I wanted that also for my children and me. Most of all I wanted freedom from Robert's emotional abuse. I wanted a normal life full of love and peace.

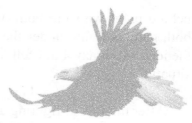

CHAPTER 22
Trying To Hold It Together

"A life of reaction is a life of slavery, intellectually and spiritually. One must fight for a life of action, not reaction."

-Rita Mae Brown

When I got home, I confronted Robert. I asked him to tell me the truth of what was really going on. He told me he was in love with someone else. They had been together for a long time. He wouldn't say how long though. I thought I was going to throw up. The worse part… I knew her, and her family. Robert was having an affair with a woman in his office, who just happened to be the niece of my father's best friend. I was stunned and totally speechless. I felt betrayed. I was such a fool. His comments about being naïve were beginning to make sense. If this wasn't a test for my stress level and this disease, I don't know what else could be. I talked and Robert avoided. To me, family and sticking together through good times and bad are very important. The disease had been very challenging, and in the past, there had been times when he had supported me. Now, with me in better health, I could be patient, learn to forgive Robert, and he would change and learn to love me again. I asked if he would change jobs, and end his affair, because that would help me to forgive him. I knew in time we could put this behind us, if we were both willing. I wanted my children to have both parents living under the same roof, and being happy. I knew the idea was crazy, but I felt in time somehow I could look past this situation.

After months of fighting and convincing Robert to change jobs, with great resistance, he did. He still continued coming home late. I thought he had a heavy work load and never gave his late hours a second thought. Once again a little too naïve and trusting. I convinced Robert to start to wear his wedding ring again, but as I watched him get into the car to leave, he took it off. He didn't see me watching. That really hurt me. I knew his words and promises were empty and would never be fulfilled. I was a big joke to Robert. I was being used. He was staying with me to see the children, and have a place to live. He was not ready to pay the costs involved with divorce.

Whenever we spoke of his affair, Robert continuously insisted that she was a very nice girl. It wasn't the sort of thing the wife wants to hear. He kept defending her which confused me and made me feel sick to my stomach. It didn't sound like he was moving forward, it sounded like he was living in the past. I continuously wondered how Robert's behavior would affect my children's future relationships.

The marriage counselor, the massage therapist, and my strong inner voice were telling me to value myself, and make the first move to end this loveless marriage, but I couldn't bring myself to do it. I was extremely fearful of what the future would hold.

I was breaking cardboard boxes down in the garage one evening. I was upset and not focusing on what I was doing. I had trouble breaking one particular box down and got frustrated. I jumped on it and began to cry. To me, it symbolized how I couldn't get anything right. I slipped and fell on my elbow fracturing it. I knew instantly something was terribly wrong. The pain was so bad;

I thought I was going to be sick to my stomach. I was very dizzy. I lay on the cement garage floor feeling I was safer there than getting up, passing out, and hitting my head. Once again, Robert was no where to be found. I got myself into the house. Lynn took one look at me and took over. She called my father.

My father took me to the hospital. The doctor confirmed my thoughts. I had fractured my elbow and needed a cast. The doctor's first question was, "Is this from domestic abuse?" I felt like crying and saying, "Yes." But, it was not obvious abuse. It was not physical abuse. The kind of abuse I suffered left no visible scars. I did not speak up. I held my secret and pain inside.

Later that evening, Robert got home. After seeing the cast, he didn't even ask what had happened. In the middle of the night, when I needed to take more Tylenol 3's for the pain, he refused to get it for me. I ended up opening the bottle with my teeth. I cried myself to sleep once again. I prayed to God to give me some answers. I needed to know why my life was so out of control. Robert was sleeping on the couch. He gave me absolutely no support. I was basically facing each new disaster alone. I laid there feeling desperate and alone. Rocky cuddled into me, I held him and realized that without his unconditional love and support I would not be able to survive.

The next week, while visiting with my mother, I was holding Marie in my arms. She was strangely quiet for a three year old. I checked her head. She was burning up with a fever. The next thing I knew she was unconscious. I called the doctor and was told to get her to the hospital immediately. I tried to phone Robert at his office. They did not know where he was. My father rushed over to our house, carried Marie to the car, and placed her against me.

When we got to the hospital, he carried Marie into the Emergency, while I answered questions for the nurse. The first question she asked was, "Where is the father?" I wanted to say,

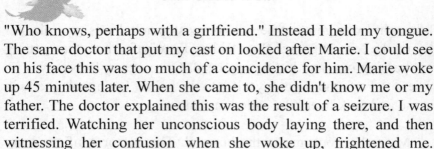

"Who knows, perhaps with a girlfriend." Instead I held my tongue. The same doctor that put my cast on looked after Marie. I could see on his face this was too much of a coincidence for him. Marie woke up 45 minutes later. When she came to, she didn't know me or my father. The doctor explained this was the result of a seizure. I was terrified. Watching her unconscious body laying there, and then witnessing her confusion when she woke up, frightened me. Fortunately within half an hour, she was back to her old self. Later that evening when Robert got home, he didn't believe a word of it.

Robert's double life was becoming too much for him to handle. His lies were weighing heavily on him. One day he came home and said he needed to get away for awhile and re-evaluate what he wanted in his life. All the time he spoke, never once did he make eye contact. I was getting exceedingly fed up with him coming home late, no communication, and no laughter in our life. I was getting fed up with him not making up his mind what he wanted or moving forward in life. I was relieved to see Robert go away for three days. I later learned it was a romantic weekend for him and his girlfriend. Was I hurt? Heck ya! I knew the marriage was over and I was going to become a statistic.

I saw how short life can be from my experiences and Marie's, and I did not want to lose another minute of my life over someone who didn't know if he wanted a wife or girlfriend.

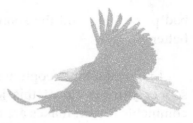

CHAPTER 23
Taking Back My Power

"Relax your mind and let your senses come alive."

-author unknown

That next week when I was having a massage I shared with the therapist what Robert had done. I cried continuously throughout my treatment. The massage therapist said, "The sooner you get rid of this jerk from your life, the better." He suggested I look at getting into regular exercise as another way to alleviate the stress. He recommended I join a gym that had just opened up in town.

This was my first time exercising in years. The trainers at the gym told me I needed permission from my family doctor. My doctor suggested I work with a trainer and learn how to do the various exercises the correct way. That would avoid injury. My personal trainer, David, was a terrific guy. A friendly outgoing guy, he was kind, spiritual, and loved by everyone. He had a great sense of humor. Working with Dave, not only helped me gain strength and tone, he also increased my confidence and was a huge boost to my self-esteem. Dave convinced me, "The comments Robert makes are out of hate and fear. He is the one with the problem, not you." Dave would continuously say, "That guy is a person living in a very bad place." He said the sooner I got rid of him from my life, the better.

I noticed many people were making the same comments. "The sooner you get rid of this jerk from your life, the better." "The comments Robert makes are out of hate and fear. He is the one with the problem, not you." With their support, I knew ending the marriage was the right thing to do. I was beginning to feel I would survive.

Over the years, each time Robert used hateful and degrading words, I would turn to food. On difficult days when I had no clue where he was, I would binge, eating everything in sight. Over a couple of years, living like this, I gained twenty pounds. However, I was taking back my power. I found the more I toned and lost weight, the better I felt about myself. My confidence and self-esteem increased tremendously. My blood work improved. I was no longer anemic. I surrounded myself with new friends. I was now involved with people who were always positive and loved life.

Dave was always great at motivating me to learn new things. He felt the more I tried new activities, the more my confidence would grow. He was right. I was scared. What if the Crohns flared up while I was doing one of these new activities? I could see myself, frantic, out in the middle of nowhere searching for a washroom. However, Dave was good! My first new activity was to learn how to roller-blade. During my illness, through my bedroom window, I had watched many people tackling what I thought, was an easy sport. After all, I had been a bronze medallist in figure skating. How hard could it be? I thought learning this new sport was going to be a breeze. Boy was I wrong.

As my confidence grew, I started going up and down hills. That is when I ran into some problems. The faster I came down those hills, the harder I landed on the pavement. Sometimes I landed face first, and sometimes I landed on my butt. I have scars to prove it.

Although I fell countless times, over and over, I felt like a winner, simply because I tried.

As the seasons changed, I picked a new activity. The next challenge was to learn cross-country skiing. I found most of it easy. However, I couldn't perfect the art of going up hill. I would get up so far, angle the skis outward, and form the V. Then, the skis would cross over each other, behind me. I would slide backwards, down the hill, eventually falling. My children thought it was the funniest thing, seeing their Mom coming down backwards, falling on her face, or landing on her butt. I never gave up, and kept persisting, until I improved. Once again I felt like a winner.

With the next new season approaching, I chose golfing. It was a terrific feeling being able to be out in nature and not have to be near a washroom. Although I was able to hit the ball, I had no control over the direction it ended up going. Every time there was a water hazard, my ball was attracted to it. I was always fishing my ball out of the ponds, creeks and miniature lakes. Golf is a challenge I am definitely still working on. I am a work in progress.

Trying new activities continued each season. The activities ranged from roller-blading; downhill skiing; golfing; and hiking to rock climbing. After I tackled a new sport or activity my confidence got stronger. I learned Crohn's disease was no longer going to hold me back. I was becoming the person I always wanted to be. I was proud of who I was, who I was becoming, and of every accomplishment.

I was receiving proof that everything happens for a reason. My inner voice had directed me to join the gym, and it had proved a great idea. I was warmly supported by other members working out, as well as from the trainers and staff. The staff even surprised me with a presentation; making me their first "Member of the Month." I was given a plaque with wonderful words about the kind person I was, always inspiring others. The card said, ATTITUDE. Attitude is a little thing that makes a BIG difference. This is the following what the plaque said. "Sue has been a member of the club since we first opened in May. Since then she has changed her life with physical fitness and her program. Sue is what we call a regular around the club always able to get her three (and often times more) workouts in each week. The best part about Sue is her enthusiasm, friendly face and her willingness to do anything she can to get involved. Sue spearheaded our Christmas Angel Tree. Knowing no details about the program or the families we were sponsoring, Sue went out on her own initiative and bought crayons and coloring books for the children on our tree. Always thinking of others, Sue treats the staff to her awesome homemade bread on a regular basis. We love that! Sue also was behind the naming of the Daycare center as the "Junior Fitness Room" and has been known to donate a bag of toys now and again. If you see Sue around the club be sure to congratulate her because she is a fantastic person to have as our friend!" This was another time in my life when it was brought to my attention that helping others was my purpose in life.

I worked out five days a week. My blood levels improved. I toned. I felt less stress. My self esteem was growing. I even won a prize for coming up with the best name for the daycare center at the gym. We called it "The Junior Fitness Room".

Even with the stress of Robert still living under the same roof, exercising and the whole atmosphere, with the positive people at the gym, helped me feel better about myself. I knew when Robert walked out; I was going to be okay. I believe, by guiding me to the gym, God and his angels were helping me prepare for the adjustment of separation and becoming a single Mom. My life would be better. I started to believe I was a much better person than Robert had been telling me for countless years.

Robert really hated seeing me happy. When I shared my award with the girls, he was not impressed. The next day he brought home a new used car, and told me it was to be my vehicle. It was an ugly gold station wagon. A week later Robert announced he was leaving. It was February 14th. On that same day fifteen years earlier he had proposed to me.

Robert left while the girls were at school. After packing his things into the car, he wrote each of the girls a letter, saying he would always be there for them. Robert angrily shouted his last words to me, "I will spend the rest of my life ruining your life, just like you ruined mine by having that disease!"

How had I missed such hate and revenge in someone I was with for over 18 years? Dave's words echoed back to me, "Robert is full of hate and fear. That is his stuff, not yours." I was shocked by the amount of hate and anger he had towards me, but remembering Dave's words brought me back into focus. It was his problem, not mine.

Watching Robert head out the door for the last time was a great relief. No longer did I have to hear his hateful words. No longer did I have to wonder when he would be home for dinner, or who he was with. This took a huge weight off my shoulders.

Later that evening, the Gastroenterologist's words echoed in the back of my mind. "This is a tough disease to cope with. Many couples don't stay together." Remembering these words I thought he was right. I worried that no man would ever want to share my life with me ever again. However, I knew that I could survive.

Not only would I survive, I would put my mind to it and thrive. I was finally free.

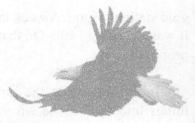

CHAPTER 24
Accepting Divorce

"The obstacles of your past can become the gateways that lead to new beginnings."

-Ralph Blum

When I shared my separation news with my personal trainer, Dave, he was relieved. He was excited for me. It was a new beginning.

My next step was to take up yoga. Dave thought this would help me cope with the stress of the divorce. Yoga was being offered at the gym. I could bring the girls with me, and they could go in the playroom. This way I didn't have to worry about the cost of a babysitter. I had decided to accept that all things came to me for a reason. I didn't want to be closed minded about anything ever again.

The brochure said, "Yoga is a form of gentle exercise for all ages consisting of body postures and breathing techniques. Yoga is a mental and physical training. Yoga is beneficial for stress, fatigue, headaches, migraines, depression, circulatory disorders, digestive disorders, back pain, and menstrual problems, including PMS.

Yoga postures develop physical flexibility and controlled relaxation to harmonize the mind, body and soul."

I had to have my doctor's permission before starting the program. To my surprise, because of having a doctor's letter, I was able to claim the cost under my medical expenses on my taxes.

Going to the first yoga class opened my eyes to all the benefits it could offer me. Yoga did help me cope with the unpleasant divorce. I found it to be calming. I was grounded and focused after a yoga session. My body became more toned. I would have to say that practicing yoga was one of the best things I have ever done for myself.

When I first started doing Yoga, my stomach got gassy. I later learned this was a healing occurring. If you have digestive disorders don't let this stop you from taking a class, just be sure and be at the back of the room, close to a washroom for the first few classes. Yoga classes lasted from a minimum of 30 minutes to 1 ½ hours. I learned that doing Yoga should never cause severe pain and should be done at your own pace. I took my time and did not push myself. I gradually increased my endurance. After the first couple of classes, I experienced slight stiffness in my joints. When this happened, I would drink plenty of water and soak in an Epsom Salt bath before bed.

The Yoga helped me. I always got renewed energy and my appetite increased after each class. My daily routine improved because of my being more focused. I enthusiastically helped out at the school. I began to enjoy gardening again and I didn't even mind cleaning the house. I even had more energy to play with the girls.

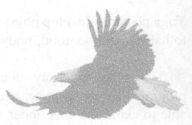

CHAPTER 25
Jumping Through The Legal Hoops

"Realize that true happiness lies within you. Waste no time and effort searching for peace and contentment and joy in the world outside. Remember that there is no happiness in having or in getting, but only in giving. Reach out. Share. Smile. Hug. Happiness is a perfume you cannot pour on others without getting a few drops on yourself."

-Og Mandino

I was one of those individuals who said, "My husband will never have an affair. Divorce will never happen to me." Never say never.

Here I was getting a divorce. I felt naïve for believing every lie Robert had ever told me. I was also scared, facing unknown changes that would powerfully affect my children's lives and my own. I was anxious about surviving financially. I worried I would be unable to repair things around our home. I was afraid that if I got sick again I might not be able to raise my children. I realized I was focusing on everything negative. From the inspirational books I was reading and comments from my personal trainer; I was aware that focusing on the negative attracts more negative. However, it was extremely hard for me to stop focusing on everything that was wrong or bad in my life.

Sitting in the darkness, alone, late at night, I turned my thoughts from the dark memories of the bad things that had happened, to feelings of gratitude for the weight that had been lifted from my shoulders. I knew that it was not going to be easy, but was relieved that the stress and tension were gone. There were times when I actually said out loud, "Thank God, it is over."

I had to concentrate on taking care of my girls, maintaining my health, and continuously moving forward. Each day I struggled to build my self-confidence, find strength from within, and learn to like myself. Over time, it got easier.

As I went through the divorce, there were obvious stages of mourning. The first stage was denial. "This can't be happening to me." I looked for Robert in familiar places. I didn't cry or even acknowledge the loss. I didn't share with people that I was going through a divorce.

The second stage was anger. I wanted to fight back or get even with him. I blamed Robert for everything. I felt he had ruined Lynn and Marie's childhood memories, been emotionally unavailable when I was sick and needed him the most and he was the cause of the divorce. Robert had lied to me, cheated on me, and abandoned the three of us. That made me very angry.

Stage three was bargaining. For the sake of the girls, I attempted to bargain for reconciliation. I said, "If I stay healthy, maybe we can make it work." Robert's only response was, "I need more time."

I bargained with God. "I promise to be a better person, if you bring Robert back." I was begging, wishing, praying for him to

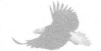

come back. "I would try harder," I constantly promised.

Stage four was depression. I had overwhelming feelings of hopelessness, frustration, bitterness, and self-pity. I was mourning the loss of hopes, dreams and plans for the future. I found myself reflecting upon the past at a time when things had been good between us. I kept searching for the exact time when Robert's feelings changed for me.

The final stage was acceptance. I accepted the loss and was determined to be independent, financially secure, and successful. I had no idea how I would do this, I just knew I would. I acknowledged that the marriage was over and accepted responsibility for my part in ending it. An incredible weight disappeared from my shoulders. I began to live life again.

My biggest challenge was supporting my children. I had no job and I had no money. Robert had planned his departure well. He left us penniless with the fridge and cupboards bare. Robert wanted to force me to let him have the girls. If I could not feed them, they would have to live with him.

The girls started asking me when we were going to buy groceries. I told them I would see if Grandpa, Robert's father, would help us out. I figured he would. In the past he and I had shared a good relationship. I called my ex father-in-law and asked if he would buy some milk and cereal for the girls. It took all the strength I had to phone him. I told him I would pay him back when I had the money.

He told me, "You created this mess, so deal with it alone."

I was shocked and speechless. What had Robert said to make him say such a thing? Apparently, this man didn't know about his son's new girlfriend. I was beginning to learn what the phrase, "She said, he said" meant.

I knew better than to talk about how rough life had been for me living with their son. I was not going to get into any battle. I hung up the phone and told the girls, "Grandpa won't help us." I sat down and cried. The girls got mad at him. They took it very personally that he would not help us out. They never had any respect for him after that.

When Robert left he took all our money, cancelled our joint credit cards, and cashed out the Air Miles points, without telling me. I had planned to buy groceries with the Air Miles points but that no longer was an option. While I was buying socks and underwear for the children, it was very embarrassing for me to learn from a Sear's store cashier, that Robert had cancelled my card. The woman behind me muttered to her friend, "That poor girl, she must be going through a divorce." I wanted to crawl under the counter. I didn't want people to know I was separated or going through a divorce.

I grew up believing families stay together no matter what. It was tough for me having to admit I was going to be a divorcee.

My parents heard the stress in my voice. They knew I had no money of my own. They asked me, "What are you going to do financially?" I was speechless. I was trying to keep myself brave for the girls. They offered to pay my legal costs and buy food for us until I got some money from Robert, or found a job, whichever came first. I didn't have any other options at this point and was grateful for their assistance.

Becoming separated and going through divorce drastically changed my life. I no longer had anything in common with friends who were married. People I thought were my friends, acted otherwise. I spent a lot of time alone reflecting on what went wrong in my marriage. When I got depressed, I went to the gym for a workout at least six days out of the week. When the girls were with their father, I wished I had friends to go to a show with. I found those weekends very difficult. It was an unpleasant feeling being alone. I had devoted all my time to my children. I no longer was interested in doing crafts or reading. I spent the weekends worrying about the girls. "Were they okay? Did they want to come home? Was their father keeping them there against their will?" Robert did not provide a phone number or his new address. The girls complained that, when Robert had them alone he was controlling. Even when I listened to him speak to them; he would talk down to them in an angry voice. They were not allowed to take their toys or stuffed animals to his home. Robert didn't want the scent of the dog or the dirt from our house to be tracked into his. All of this made me feel incredibly helpless. How could I protect my girls?

I knew that I needed to create a new beginning with Robert. So, when he called one day, to say he knew I had a massage appointment and he wanted to know if it was okay for him to stay at the house and look after the girls instead of me getting a babysitter, I thought it would be fine. I wanted the girls to have their father in their life.

I returned from my appointment and Robert quickly left. While I was cleaning up, I noticed some areas of the house were unorganized and messy. The house looked different. I was curious and questioned the girls.

They told me their father had been going through different areas of the house, taking stuff, and putting it in a garbage bag. They said Robert told them not to tell me what he had done. This upset me. It certainly sounded like he wanted them to cover up for something he shouldn't have been doing. I knew that Robert had removed some of our things. I was not certain what was missing. There were toys, pictures and other household items missing. I felt Robert was being sneaky and dishonest, and I wanted the relationship with him over. He had sounded sincere and ready to help with the girls. His words invoked a picture of cooperation and friendliness but his actions proved otherwise.

One particular day at the gym, I ran into a woman who was the mother of a friend of Lynn's. Her name was Carol. At first glance, I thought she looked terrible. She shared with me how she wasn't doing too well. Carol's husband had just walked out on her. Carol said he left her for a woman who was a grandmother. That didn't go over too well. Carol was questioning her looks and finding personal faults. I shared my story with her. Although she was sorry for me, it made her feel better that she was not alone. I agreed. I was glad that I was not going to be alone. I told her my separation was very new. I was looking for direction. I had no idea where to start when it came to divorce. Robert had filled my head with confusing information. He threatened to take the girls and leave me destitute. It didn't sound right but I didn't know what to believe.

I told Carol that my parents were helping me financially. She informed me that it was the children's father's responsibly to provide for them. She gave me the phone number for her lawyer.

Robert's suspicious actions and my fears gave me the strength to call the lawyer the next day. I realized that I needed to finalize the separation, proceed with the divorce, and end the struggle.

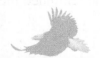

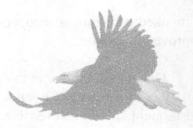

CHAPTER 26
Life Goes On

"If you're going to seek revenge you'd better dig two graves."
-Old Chinese Proverb

I was blessed to have Barb, my new lawyer, come into my life. There aren't many lawyers like this woman. I will never forget our first appointment. I was nervous and scared, afraid to hear what she had to say.

She said, "If you ever do anything that is dishonest, I will make you accountable. I don't want that karma coming back to me." She assured me that everything Robert had done would come back on him in time. If it didn't happen in this lifetime, then it would happen in another one. I have to tell you, this gave me great comfort. I did want rotten things to happen to him.

I was ready to go the legal route. I wanted the truth to come out. People needed to see the real him. The person I had hidden from everyone for so long. Robert had given me misinformation. Barb cleared it up. I was entitled to alimony, medical benefits, and child support from Robert. I told her, that Robert didn't want me to go to a lawyer. He said we could settle this ourselves. She reminded me

Robert had not been honest in years. I should not start believing him now. Barb said Robert knew he would have to pay support. He was trying to get out of it. She explained that divorce proceedings could become very difficult and nasty. She suggested I leave our meeting, absorb what she had said, and if I wanted to proceed, give her a call.

I left that meeting with mixed emotions. I felt confident Barb would help me sort this all out and get closure, but I was scared. Where would I find the money for groceries, clothes for the girls, and the lawyer's bill?

I called Barb a couple of days later. I told her that my parents had to support the girls and me, because there was no money coming from Robert. She was furious. I complained that Robert would promise to give me money, but when he came to pick up the girls for a visit, I would ask, "Do you have the money?" Robert would just smile and say, "I don't think so."

We hung up the phone and she booked a court date to have Robert's wages garnisheed.

The morning of the court case, I reflected back to my last trip to court, when I had to testify regarding the car accident. This time, I didn't want to do anything stupid or embarrassing. My lawyer, Barb, met me and my parents in the cafeteria. She said she wanted to keep me calm. We didn't want to upset my health. She said she would be in the courtroom representing me; I would stay in the cafeteria; and she would come to me during the time when I had to agree or disagree. I liked the set up. She had thought of everything. She kept me calm, by a washroom, and by food when I needed it. It was a long morning. My mind was going a mile a minute. I watched people coming and going from the cafeteria. They appeared fearful and highly emotional. Some were crying. Some were screaming at their lawyers. It was not a pleasant atmosphere. After three hours, she returned with a smile on her face. "You can

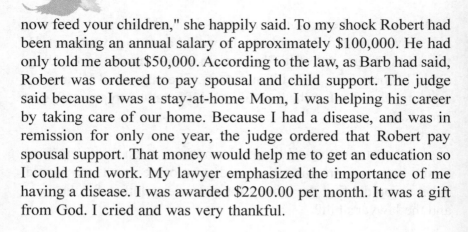

now feed your children," she happily said. To my shock Robert had been making an annual salary of approximately $100,000. He had only told me about $50,000. According to the law, as Barb had said, Robert was ordered to pay spousal and child support. The judge said because I was a stay-at-home Mom, I was helping his career by taking care of our home. Because I had a disease, and was in remission for only one year, the judge ordered that Robert pay spousal support. That money would help me to get an education so I could find work. My lawyer emphasized the importance of me having a disease. I was awarded $2200.00 per month. It was a gift from God. I cried and was very thankful.

Angered by losing control, and having to pay me money, Robert started to harass me. He would sit in front of my house in his car until I phoned the police to escort him away. Robert had decided he didn't have to follow any schedule; he would come and go as he pleased. I found letters in my mailbox which he had dropped off before seven a.m. I had countless phone calls where the phone would ring and when I picked it up, nobody was there. When I shared this with my lawyer, she said the only way to stop him from sitting in front of the house was to go to court and get a court order setting up a regular schedule for visitation. Because Robert was sitting on a public street, the police couldn't charge him. If they felt he was harassing me, they could escort him away.

She suggested I call and report his actions to the police every time. She didn't get a good feeling about this man. She said by making a police report, it would show his patterns of harassment if things got worse. She told me to avoid being anywhere alone. She was worried what else Robert might try.

Throughout the entire process, my lawyer didn't tell me Robert was going for sole custody. She knew if I knew this it would devastate me. She was right. For eight months we went through a clinical/ psychological assessment. The Psychologist, appointed by the courts, observed the children playing with each of us separately. He noted that Robert did not play naturally with the children. He made them sit and do math work. Robert even yelled at Lynn telling her to 'shut up'. He knew he was being watched, and his actions and words truly illustrated what kind of a man he really was.

One of Lynn's teachers shared with me how his sister had gone through a similar custody battle. He said the best defense for me is to have people who knew us simply tell the Psychologist the truth, and share their comments on our parenting. I found it difficult to ask people to share their comments. Someone, I still don't know who, started getting friends and family to write testimonial letters on my behalf and gave them to my lawyer. Barb shared 64 positive letters. People praised me for how I always put my children first, in spite of the disease.

The week before the hearing for the final decision, my lawyer then shared with me the fact that Robert was going for sole custody. I was shocked and heartbroken. I thought this was a hearing regarding where the children would live. Never did it occur to me that I could possibly lose visitation rights to my own children. My children meant the world to me. I didn't want to lose them. Robert was trying to prove that anyone with Crohns disease was not a fit parent.

When I heard my lawyer say that Robert was going for sole custody, and heard his reason, I was even more determined to keep healthy. Barb recommended I go away for the weekend before the hearing and just rest. She wanted me to be calm, rested, and healthy-looking.

Taking her advice, a girlfriend and I went to a spa resort for the weekend. When we checked in, we were given a cozy robe to wear all weekend. We enjoyed healing treatments of Reiki, Reflexology, and meditation. We ate all natural food by a cozy fireplace. It was the best medicine for me to prepare for an unknown fate that I was not sure I could handle.

Before going to the meeting, I prayed to God to have the Psychologist make the right decision. I knew what Robert had put me through, and I didn't want to see my children go through the same routine of abuse and hate. My lawyer assured me, "It will be okay. You are a terrific mother and a wonderful person." She was my rock. After her reassuring words, I went into the hearing feeling confident that the judge would make the right decision. I was a terrific mother, and I was determined to never get sick again.

I felt he knew our true personalities. I was right. The Psychologist said, "After reading those touching letters, I know that if you ever get sick again, you will be well supported." He ordered Robert to take a course in parenting skills, "Something he was lacking tremendously," the Psychologist shared. You have never seen such a grateful mother anywhere as I was that day.

Robert got up, yelled at the Psychologist, threw papers around the room, and then he stormed out. After Robert left the Psychologist said he felt it was best for my lawyer and I to stay in his office to give Robert some time to leave the area. The Psychologist was concerned that Robert might harm me. I too, was frightened and relieved that he said to stay. Robert's sneakiness and lies had finally caught up with him. Although, a part of me was sympathetic and felt sorry for him, I was pleased that the girls would be protected from his constant influence. The Psychologist's decision was a good one.

I hugged Barb, thanking her for saving my children from a terrible fate. I hugged the Psychologist, telling him how grateful I was for his decision. I cried, knowing in my heart that I was now totally responsible, and also knowing that I could do it.

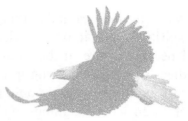

CHAPTER 27
Not All Sunny Skies

"Man often becomes what he believes himself to be. If I keep on saying to myself that I cannot do a certain thing, it is possible that I may end by really becoming incapable of doing it. On the contrary, if I shall have the belief that I can do it, I shall surely acquire the capacity to do it, even if I may not have it at the beginning."

-Mahatma Gandhi

It was comforting having Carol in my life at that time. We helped each other through difficult days. We shared the same schedule. Our children were with their respective fathers at the same time. We would meet at the gym in the mornings, come back to my place for lunch, and go to a movie in the evening. We would talk, and complain, and support each other. We understood each other. We focused on enjoying life. We laughed more, and began to do new things. We started going to movies that our husbands would never go to, "chick flicks." It was fun going to shows where the other person didn't complain through it.

I made a conscious decision to enjoy being outdoors more. I spent time cutting the grass, and doing the gardening. Instead of watching movies and staying in the house, I took a 'self-help' or 'spiritual' book into the backyard, and sat in the warmth of the sun. I became aware of the sounds of nature. The birds were singing, there were dogs barking in the neighborhood, and the leaves were rustling in the wind. I could hear the voices of people near by, and children were laughing and playing. I no longer focused on the negative in my life. I was now seeing and hearing a whole new world.

I began to look at life in a positive way. I started to believe the comments of the marriage counselor. "There are other men out there." "You are pretty." "You are strong. You have survived a lot already." One of my biggest fears had been that I would be alone. I now realized that I was contented, even when alone. I was becoming my own person, and for now that was enough.

It was actually nice not to have to ask someone for permission. I liked making my own decisions. I could purchase a new pair of socks, makeup, or clothing, without giving an explanation. I could go to lunch with a friend, get a massage, or get my hair done without an argument. I had my own vehicle and could come and go as I please. There was a wonderful sense of freedom.

I followed a routine of going to the gym, eating healthy, and reading positive books. I did everything in my power to maintain a great attitude. I found the people at the gym to be beyond friendly. They were positive, encouraging, and overwhelmingly supportive. There were times when I would enter the building and immediately be drawn aside by one of the personal trainers. They had noticed, by the look on my face, that I was having a difficult day. We went into one of the consulting rooms, and they used words of encouragement to give me strength. "You are a good person." "You can get through this." "You have the strength to cope." Their comforting words would evoke a torrent of tears. Often this was the release I needed.

The tension in the house was better and my health had improved. I was more relaxed and able to create a stable home for the girls. They attended the nearby school, we cooked meals together, and we read stories at bedtime. At the end of the day I asked them, "What was the best part of your day?" I wanted them to concentrate on the positive.

Because of my improved health, I was able to do more things with the girls. They delighted in playing baseball with me in the backyard, my attempts at skiing, and picking me up when I fell at rollerblading. I focused on them. We purchased an above-ground pool for the backyard and laughed and played for hours. I was a big kid. The housework was left until dark and fun was the priority.

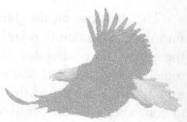

CHAPTER 28
Peace and Possibilities

"It is hard to soar like an eagle when you are surrounded by turkeys."
-Unknown Author

The children were expected to go with Robert on Wednesday nights and every other weekend. As time passed, more and more often, he called to say, "Something has come up, and I can't pick you up for our weekly visit." It was difficult for me to sit back and watch the pain on their faces. This emotional abuse hurt all of us. I started having headaches, pains in my neck, and severe aches in my stomach. I was unaware of how much this situation really bothered me until friends pointed it out. They would tell me I had to let go and let God look after this situation, or it would kill me. I started reading books where those exact words, "Let go and let God," would stand out on pages. I even borrowed a book, "Conversations with God", where a friend had underlined for herself the exact phrase "Let go and let God take over this situation". Talk about a Higher Power giving me a message. Many friends told me the same thing. After a very long time, too long, I managed to take these words to heart.

The first Christmas was extremely difficult. The girls were scheduled to go to their father's at noon on Christmas Eve and be returned to my place by noon on Christmas day. Traditionally, Christmas Eve and morning were important to us. We had always made a fuss about leaving milk and cookies for Santa. For me to be home alone was devastating. My parents had picked up my Grandmother and, as was their yearly routine, were spending Christmas Eve with friends. I stayed home alone, watching rented movies while eating a toasted peanut butter and jam sandwich.

The children didn't like being away from home for that first Christmas. After dinner on Christmas Eve, they asked to be brought back home. Robert refused to bring them. He said, "It is my time." Marie, at the age of five, was not one to speak out, instead she acted out. She took the scissors, and cut off one of her nice long blonde braided pony tails. Marie didn't like the changes to her routine. She didn't like the lack of control in her life.

When Marie was returned on Christmas day, she was wearing a hat and refused to take it off. When she did remove it, I was shocked and appalled at the sight of her hair. Half of her hair was literally chopped off, uneven, and it would be months before it was presentable. It was so bad that I didn't want to attempt to fix it. When my parents came to the door, I met them, and whispered, "Marie chopped her hair off, don't say a word." Knowing how upset the children were, we avoided talking about the situation. On Boxing Day, the girls and I spent the day with Carol and her children at her house. She had experience in hairdressing. She did her best to fix Marie's hair.

When I learned my children were going to have a step-mother, it was very difficult for me to handle. At first she bought them gifts. I could not buy extravagant gifts, nor did I want to. The girls, of course, liked getting these gifts. For a short while, they looked forward to going with Robert, just to see what they would get next. The insecure side of me thought I was losing them.

121

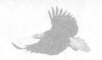

Lynn noticed how I became quiet whenever she and Marie spoke of the step-mother. I chanced being hurt more, and shared how I felt. They both assured me she would never replace me. Even though Robert insisted that they call her Mom, they never would. The girls and their friends called her, "Barbie." Marie said, "Mommy, my friends say she looks like Barbie. She is always getting her hair and nails done." Lynn said, "She is really high maintenance."

One day while out for a walk in the park, I came across a heart-wrenching scene. Right in front of my path stood Robert with his arm around his girlfriend. She was holding my youngest daughter in her arms, and Lynn was standing by Robert. If one didn't know, you'd think they were a happy family. Robert had a smirk on his face. He was smiling, knowing the pain the scene was causing me. His girlfriend looked uncomfortable. I didn't say a word; I turned off the sidewalk, rushed to my car, and went home and cried for the rest of the day. I couldn't get the scene out of my head. I prayed Robert would one day feel that same pain and hurt.

They were not a happy family. There were many times when Robert only took Marie because he and Lynn were not getting along. Lynn was angry at his lies, and she blamed Robert for the breakup of our family. Robert did not allow the girls to bring any of their gifts from him home, and they were not allowed to bring their toys with them when they visited. Robert refused their request to have a pet at his house. The tension grew between them. Eventually, the children were not welcome in his home. When Robert had time with the girls, he would take them to a hotel to avoid conflict between him and his girlfriend.

Just days after our divorce was final, Robert married his girlfriend. He did not tell the girls of the marriage until weeks later. They were hurt and upset by this.

Robert actually had the nerve to call me and insisted that I help him convince the girls to like his new wife and call her, "Mom". He went on to say his wife didn't like the girls, and they didn't like her. I smiled inside. I was glad to hear life was not going perfectly for Robert. What did he expect? How did Robert think the girls would feel not being included in his wedding? I refused to help him in his effort to 'control' the girls. Instead, I said, "I am sorry to hear that."

As I smiled looking towards God, I thanked Robert for being who he was, and for teaching me many valuable lessons in life. He was speechless. I told Robert when one is deceitful, it always has a way of coming back on you. I told him it was a lesson I hoped he learned one day for the sake of our children. Robert told me how he had a plan on how his life would be and it was not turning out at all like he wanted. Once again, I looked up towards heaven and said, "Thank you."

Some people become resentful towards the opposite sex, when abuse or betrayal occurs. I, on the other hand, do not carry any bad feelings. I am not angry for what Robert said, or did to me, and see the entire experience as a learning lesson. I know how much strength it took for me to cope with the hurt and lies. Knowing this, I appreciate that putting my mind to something, having a positive attitude, and not holding a grudge, allows me to survive and heal.

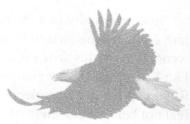

CHAPTER 29
Confident, Poised and Powerful

"You can't just sit there and wait for people to give you that golden dream. You've got to get out there and make it happen for yourself."

-Diana Ross

Because babysitting was familiar to me, I signed up again with the daycare center I worked for years ago. My home was inspected, then, children were assigned to come to my home. I had a total of seven children every day and I had requested that they be the same age as my children. It was great to have some of my own money coming in again.

We had fun; going to the library for programs, parks for picnics, and doing crafts in the backyard. I believe that children need lots of fresh air; therefore, we ate as many meals as possible outside. Sports were a big part of our day. The parents were thrilled with our routine, and my children were delighted to have me active in their day.

When all seven children attended school fulltime, I wanted a job to fill the hours while they were in school. I had gone back to volunteering once a week in my children's classes, however, I wanted more. One day, in a conversation with the principal, I mentioned my desire to be doing more, and making money at it. He had an idea.

Because of my many hours of volunteer experience at the school, and the additional hours doing daycare in my home, he felt I could qualify to teach nursery school. He wrote a powerful, extremely complimentary letter of recommendation, glowing about my accomplishments. He said, I was terrific with the children, and he thought I would make a wonderful teacher.

At the first opportunity I forwarded the letter to the director of the daycare center. Within the week, she offered me a position teaching at their nursery school. I was terrified. Once again, just like back in elementary school, I would be the center of attention. The children were between the ages of three and four, and I was afraid of them. Talk about being insecure. I knew I had to face this fear. For me, at this time in my life, it was a huge struggle, one that I was willing to face. Every time the other teacher asked me to read the story at circle time, I opted out, and chose to prepare the snacks, and clean up instead. I started with two mornings per week. As more opportunities opened up, I gratefully accepted the new positions and increased hours. My confidence grew as both parents and fellow workers showed me their appreciation, and gave me such positive feedback.

One of the activities that I looked forward to each week was the inter-generational program we ran in our local senior's home. The parents brought their toddlers in to play with the resident seniors. I enjoyed watching the children, as they laughed and played, and brought smiles to the seniors' faces. I worked with a great partner. We shared our ups and downs, and developed a great friendship.

Lynn was now in grade seven, and she wanted to attend the monthly "Much Music" Dances. When asked to volunteer as a chaperone, I accepted the challenge. This was a big step for me. I would be walking into a social setting on my own. Once again, facing a fear, with a positive attitude, I was rewarded with the satisfaction of surviving.

Although my life wasn't peaceful yet, there were signs of the possibility. I was having fun working with the children, and for the first time, socializing on my own. My confidence was building as I developed a career, and independently handled my finances.

After working in this field for a couple years, I found I wanted more freedom to be there for my children. I missed going on school trips, and volunteering in their classes. I missed meeting and getting to know their friends. I wanted to observe their progress throughout the year. I felt disconnected from that part of their life.

It was around this time, that I ran into an old school friend, someone I actually knew from kindergarten. During our catch-up conversation, he told me that he was trained in various alternative healing therapies. This intrigued me. It turned out he was taking a refresher course in Reiki just a few weeks later. I was looking for a new career, one that would give me more daytime hours for my children. In the past, I was fascinated by how Reiki helped me heal. I now decided not to ignore this new door opening up for me. I would take the training.

During the Reiki training, I learned a lot about myself. I came to terms with all that had happened in my past; childhood disappointments, the illnesses, and everything with Robert. It helped me to trust in life, knowing that everything happens for a reason. I understood the feeling of peace as it was revealed during the Reiki meditations and quiet times. I was actually beginning to feel some contentment. This training was a very powerful experience for me. At the end of the course my teacher took me aside, and told me that I had a special gift for healing. She said, "You are about to take a different path in your life." That was fine with me. I no longer feared the unknown, a new me was beginning to appear!

A year later, I was introduced to Reflexology. This is a treatment that is performed on feet, hands, and less commonly on ears. When the practitioner pressed on specific areas on my foot, it triggered reactions and healing in a particular, related body part. For example; the tips of the toes relate to the head; the ball of the foot relates to the lungs; and the heel relates to the pelvis. Often, a sense of peace and well-being permeates the body after a session. For me, muscles that were tight going into the session became loose and relaxed.

I learned Reflexology is beneficial for high blood pressure, stress, anxiety, insomnia, migraines, asthma, sinusitis, back pain, pain relief, and menstrual problems. I found this modality to be relaxing and grounding for me. It was especially helpful for my sinuses.

As a result of being so impressed by Reflexology, I studied and trained through the Ontario College of Reflexology, and became a Certified Reflexologist. I started the course in the classroom setting, then reverted to doing the course by correspondence, to accommodate the girls scheduling. They were still too young to leave alone after school. Once again, the instructor told me I was a natural healer.

After completing the Reiki and Reflexology training, I took a giant step and gave my notice to the daycare center. I opened my own Reiki/ Reflexology practice in my home. I had clients even driving four or more hours to come for my treatments. It was a wonderful feeling to help others, plus, I could make my own hours and be there for my children. My clients constantly said, "You are such an inspiration to me. I feel very motivated listening to you." I had no idea what I had said that motivated them and inspired them.

The praise continued, and people actually said that I helped them change their lives. "Changed their lives!"??? I still was confused. However, their words were about to change my future. A new door was opening.

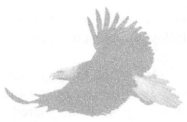

CHAPTER 30
My Earthly Angel

"Fear knocked at the door, faith answered, and no one was there."
-Old Irish Proverb

A phone call came from my Reiki teacher asking me to help a friend of hers. She wanted to introduce me to a man by the name of Lloyd Oliver. He was an intuitive counselor that was starting up a new practice. She wanted Lloyd to practice by giving me a reading.

I thought it would be just one reading. That is what I thought. He would become an earthly angel for me.

Lloyd called. Our first conversation was amazing. I felt like I had just reconnected with an old, lost friend. We set up a time to get together and have the session. I sensed that this was to be a friendship that would last a lifetime.

I had many physic readings in the past, however, nothing like the session with Lloyd. With the words he used, he was counseling me and kicking my butt to accept the power within me. Although Lloyd saw everything that lay before my path, he didn't share it all at once. He told me my strengths and weaknesses, and what steps to take next. The more I questioned him, the more he pushed me to follow through on his current advice. Then he would give me more.

One of the things I shared with Lloyd was that I was afraid of spending the rest of my life alone, never having love in my life. When I pushed, he shared details of what the man of my future would be like. He said, "He will be loved by everyone. He will be a kind man, very gentle, and older than you". When Lloyd told me the man was older, I said he was wrong. No way would I ever get involved with someone older. All through school I only dated guys my age. I was not going to start doing it now. Each similar conversation, Lloyd would simply smile and say no more.

He tried for a very long time to convince me to go to Toastmasters, an international association of clubs that help people to improve their presentation and leadership skills. I had a major fear of speaking in public. I was stubborn and did not want to face this fear. They meet once a week and most people continue for years. I did not want to be the center of attention every week.

He also asked me to start journaling everything I was going through in my life. He told me that would make things easier for me in years to come. I started and stopped and started again. I didn't see a point in writing, and he wouldn't share the reason. When he gave me suggestions over business, Reiki and Reflexology, I followed up on it immediately. When he suggested I contact a certain person, I did, and doors opened for me. It reinforced my belief in him.

The more I resisted going to Toastmasters, the more he brought it up. He was persistent, and I was stubborn. I am sure Lloyd must have asked for help from above.

One day while out shopping and running errands, I ran into a lady. A year earlier, I had given support to her and her husband, who was coping with Crohn's disease. Diane and I ran into each other several times that day. Finally, the seventh time, she mentioned, "This is very strange." We wondered why this was happening. I told Diane a friend had been kicking my butt, big time, to get me to a club called, Toastmasters. I had finally decided to go, and couldn't find their phone number. Later that evening, Diane phoned me with the number for the president of the Milton Toastmasters Club. I had no excuse not to go now. Perhaps that was our only reason for meeting. It was 'meant to be'.

A few days later, I got up the nerve, and dialed the number. I reached an answering machine. The man's voice was kind and he was soft-spoken. I left a detailed message. Three days later, Ross, called me back sounding quite puzzled at how I had gotten his cell number. Ross told me he was actually the Past- President, and his cell phone number had never been listed anywhere. After talking for about an hour, he invited me to come to a Toastmaster's meeting as his guest the following night. I accepted.

Walking through the door, for the first Toastmasters meeting, I knew instantly who Ross was. I felt comfortable around him and trusted him. He reminded me of my Grandpa Buck. Not only did he share his name but also body shape. In fact, I thought of my Grandpa Buck, while I was talking to this kind man. During our phone conversation, I had mentioned to Ross, that I had been invited to go on a local TV show. I was to be interviewed about a fundraiser I had organized. He could hear the panic in my voice. Ross volunteered to be my mentor. He said he would help me get over my fear of public speaking. He assured me I would feel more confident in no time. I told him, "You have your hands full, and your work cut out for you!"

The second Toastmasters meeting was September 11, 2001; a day that changed America, and affected millions around the world. It was a day, people will never forget. The terrible disaster in New York and Washington reminded me how short life can be. One never knows when their time will be up. This particular meeting

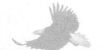

was dedicated to sharing inspirational quotes and thoughts. Ross encouraged me to share a motivational thought. I walked up to the podium feeling sick to my stomach, weak at the knees, and extremely dizzy. I focused on inspiring everyone sitting in front of me. Surprisingly, it felt great to see people smile as I spoke. I could see by their expressions, they were truly affected by my words. For the first time, I knew my words were making a positive difference for these people.

They let me know, they felt the same way, by volunteering me to give a positive thought or tip of the day at the next meeting. I loved doing that role. With the help of Ross' gentle pushes, at my third meeting I delivered my first speech. Toastmasters designed the first speech, "The Ice Breaker", to allow people to introduce themselves and speak before the group. As I delivered the speech, "Journey Towards Healing," I was amazed at how intent everyone was listening to my story. After the meeting, many shared how I had inspired them. They said they would look at life differently now. "Wow!" I thought. My words affected people that much. It amazed me. After that first speech, I was excited to share more thoughts and motivate the group weekly. I volunteered, without Ross having to nudge me.

All this time, I was sharing with Lloyd what was happening in my life since joining Toastmasters. He would only grin and tell me to keep going. I knew there was more that he was not sharing.

Because of going to Toastmasters, I had to write speeches and collect thoughts to deliver each week. I never realized how much I enjoyed writing before. Now I saw why Lloyd thought it would be good for me to be journaling. I discovered my confidence and self-esteem was growing. I looked forward to going to the weekly meetings. Not only to inspire the group, but also to learn more from Ross, and make him proud of his student.

After doing my first and second speech, public speaking got

easier. While doing my third speech, "Speaking With Sincerity", I was hit with a funny feeling; an overwhelming feeling of sadness. The speech was about Rocky and all the wonderful things he had done over his lifetime for me. As I was giving the speech, it hit me I was delivering Rocky's eulogy, and I started to get teary eyed. I noticed that everyone in the room was wiping their eyes and were very touched by my words. I turned that speech into an article and read it over and over. This was helping me prepare for his inevitable death.

A few weeks after giving that speech, I met Mark Victor Hansen, co-author of "Chicken Soup for the Soul". I shared Rocky's story with him. He read it, gave me a huge hug, and said I needed to do much more with this story. I was inspired! I went on to complete my CTM- Competent Toastmaster Award. No longer was I fearful of speaking in public. My mentor, Ross, was proud.

Our friendship was growing rapidly. I felt safe being around Ross. He was such a kind man. In every new conversation, we shared more and more about ourselves. It was incredible how much we had in common. We both loved to travel. We both had dogs.

Both of us were surprised to discover that his grandmother's name was Suzie, and my grandfather's name was Ross. We found this very eerie. At this point, I learned that Ross was five years older than me. My angel, Lloyd, had been right about many things.

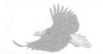

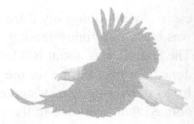

CHAPTER 31
What If He Is Mr. Right?

"I will not let my past govern my future, I shall follow my heart."
-Stephen Cotterell

Early October, I received an email from Ross. He was asking me out on a date. I was thrown off guard. I knew we were friends, however I never thought about dating. I had been focusing on my new Reiki/ Reflexology practice. When I got Ross' email I didn't know what to reply back to him. I was afraid if I went out with him, I would not focus as much on my practice. I wasn't sure if I wanted a relationship. I was starting to like being alone. I liked who I was becoming.

After a phone call to my Reiki teacher, she suggested I be open to the idea of going out with Ross. She said, "What if he is Mr. Right?" That got me thinking. He was a very kind and gentle man who I enjoyed being around. There was still that five year age difference and it kept hounding me. What if he wanted more from the relationship than I did? I didn't want to see our friendship ruined. So, I ignored the email. I didn't know what to say. After three weeks of not talking about his email when I saw him, I made a decision to go out with him. The poor guy was very relieved. He thought, when I had not brought the email up in conversation, he had crossed the line.

I was very nervous getting ready for our first date. I had planned the date for a weekend when I didn't have my girls. I didn't want them to think I was going to marry this man just because I was having dinner with him. Ross picked me up for our first date looking incredibly handsome in a suit and tie. He was taking me to a dinner theatre. Because it was a buffet, I was worried about how I would react to the food. I knew if the buffet had MSG in the food, I would react badly. I knew Ross was okay with me only drinking bottled water, therefore I didn't feel judged when I didn't order an alcoholic drink.

After dinner, I did have to run off to the washroom. The MSG had triggered a reaction in my stomach. At first I panicked, saying things to myself like: "How long am I going to be in here?" "What is Ross going to think?" "How do I stop this?" I made a decision and was determined to enjoy the evening and not let it get in my way. I started Reiki on my stomach. I continued the Reiki during the performance to calm the cramps.

I really liked spending time with Ross. It was so easy to talk to him. Our conversation never stopped. This was new for me, quality conversation with a man.

Going to this dinner theatre was a "meant to be" for me. Once the play started, I couldn't believe what I was hearing. Talk about a coincidence. It was about a married man who was having an affair. The scene played out exactly how my life had been. My first thought was, "Oh great, this cannot be happening!" As I watched, I felt no personal connection to how the wife in the play was feeling. In fact, I was grateful that Robert had done what he had done, giving me the opportunity to be here tonight, enjoying such a wonderful evening. I was happy I had accepted Ross' invitation. From that date on we saw each other almost every day and would talk for long periods of time on the phone. It was like we were kids again.

On November, 23rd, my birthday, I opened my door to a delivery man with a huge bouquet of long stemmed yellow roses. They were my favorite flowers. The birthday card attached was signed, "Love, Your secret admirer." Ross had thoughtfully respected my wish to keep our relationship quiet from the girls, until we knew where it was going. After the girls saw the card, countless questions started and didn't stop for weeks. The girls wanted to see me happy with a wonderful man in my life.

Our relationship continued in private. We talked on the phone and went hiking when the girls were with their father. We would go out for lunch when the girls were in school, and he would pick me up to drive me to the Toastmaster meetings.

In spite of our growing confidence in the relationship, I did not want to have Ross meet the girls until we were completely sure of where things were going.

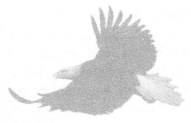

CHAPTER 32
Goodbye Rocky

"The bravest thing you can do when you are not brave is to profess courage and act accordingly."

-Corra May Harris

I watched Rocky's health deteriorate. It seemed that as my relationship with Ross grew, Rocky was able to let go. Ross was his replacement. Rocky was having trouble walking up and down stairs. He could no longer jump up onto my bed. Many mornings I would wake up to a mess on the floor. Rocky seemed to be vomiting more each day. The end of November, I made the appointment to take Rocky out of his pain and suffering. At the last minute I backed out. I was selfish. I was not ready to lose my best friend. Lloyd knew the pain I was suffering and suggested I write a list of all the good things that Rocky had done for me. That list became a speech.

When I did that speech for Toastmasters, I titled it, "The Power of Love- A Tribute to Rocky." It was the act of delivering the speech that gave me the courage to do the right thing. I knew I had to help my friend. Throughout the years he had helped me through my pain, now I had to have the courage to end his pain. After many

137

hours with Lloyd on the phone, and crying continuously in Ross' arms, I made the decision. I had Ross call the Vet to come to give Rocky 'the final needle' in the comfort of our own home. The girls said their goodbyes to Rocky the night before, and were sent off to my parents for a sleepover. I wanted some final moments alone with Rocky.

On December 3rd, the Vet came to our home. Ross placed one loving arm around me, and with the other arm he held Molly. Molly sensing what was going to happen to her friend Rocky was ready to attack the Vet and had to be restrained. I held Rocky in my arms. I wanted Rocky to feel my love while he passed. The Vet informed me what he was about to do. He would give Rocky two needles. The Vet prepared me, "We could possibly see Rocky's body spasm uncontrollably as he is dying." I panicked at the thought and began to cry uncontrollably. I didn't think I could let Rocky go. I didn't know how I could live my life without him. Both the Vet and Ross assured me I was doing the right thing for my friend. Between sobs, I kissed Rocky on the top of his head, told him, "I love you, and I will always love you." I thanked him for all the support and love he had given me in my life. I held my breath as Rocky was given the first injection. After the first needle, Rocky took one last breath and went limp. The Vet told me because I was able to let Rocky go, Rocky had passed peacefully in my arms. At 9:40 a.m. I sat on my sofa holding Rocky while wailing uncontrollably. Although, Rocky was no longer with us I didn't want to let him out of my arms. I didn't want the Vet to take him that last time.

Ross let Molly sniff Rocky one last time for her to say her goodbyes. She laid her head on Rocky's body and laid there whimpering loudly. It was heart breaking, watching her actions and hearing her pain. I had not expected her to be affected like I was. Feeling her pain and loss, Ross and I both broke into more tears. The Vet wrenched Rocky out of my arms, wrapped him in a blanket, and took him out the front door. I am sure my wails of pain could be heard a block away. For weeks, Molly stayed in the front hall area. She was waiting for her friend to return. She and I suffered the loss of Rocky for a very long time. We comforted each other and helped each other cope.

Just before Rocky died, magazines in three different countries; Canada, the United States, and England; had picked up Rocky's story, "The Power of Love- A Tribute to Rocky." I had kept in touch with the editors and shared how my furry friend had passed on. Many of them published a memorial in their magazines with a short story of how animals come into our lives at a time when we really need them. To my surprise, I started receiving sympathy cards from many people. One kind lady sent me an angel dog pin which I wear to every event I do. I also received this touching poem from many people, Rainbow Bridge. It gave me a sense of peace and helped me cope.

Rainbow Bridge

Just this side of heaven is a place called Rainbow Bridge.

When an animal dies that has been especially close to someone here, that pet goes to Rainbow Bridge.

There are meadows and hills for all of our special friends so they can run and play together.

There is plenty of food, water, and sunshine, and our friends are warm and comfortable.

All the animals that had been ill and old are restored to health and vigor.

Those who were hurt or maimed are made whole and strong again, just as we remember them in our dreams of days and times gone by.

The animals are happy and content, except for one small thing; they each miss someone very special to them, who had to be left behind.

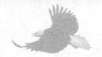

They all run and play together, but the day comes when one suddenly stops and looks into the distance.

His bright eyes are intent. His eager body quivers.

Suddenly, he begins to run from the group, flying over the green grass, his legs carrying him faster and faster.

You have been spotted, and when you and your special friend finally meet, you cling together in joyous reunion, never to be parted again.

The happy kisses rain upon your face; your hands again caress the beloved head, and you look once more into the trusting eyes of your pet, so long gone from your life but never absent from your heart.

Then you cross Rainbow Bridge together.
- *Anonymous*

In life everything happens for a reason. In my life I was given a dog named Rocky to get me through many very difficult days. He passed away at a time when he knew I would be okay without him at my side. He passed away after my doctor told me I had only 1 % chance of ever getting sick again, and just after my soul mate, Ross, came into my life to take his place. Rocky showed me I had unknown strength to survive many challenges. He gave me determination I didn't know I had.

Later that week, while crying in Ross' arms the song, "Hero", came on the radio. Ross turned to me and said, "Sue, let me be your hero." He wanted to take Rocky's place. I allowed it. I am sure it was also Rocky's wish.

We all miss Rocky very much and I thank God for all the time I have had with my magnificent friend. All those years earlier I rescued Rocky from being put down at a young age. Never did I expect he would save my life many times over. Rocky's memory will live with me eternally. Not a day passes when I don't think of him. His blue collar with his brass heart tag hangs on my bed post and before I go to sleep at night I smile and send my furry friend lots of love. Occasionally Molly will sniff his collar and then lay against me asking for cuddles. I have had some nights where the heart tag will rattle against the bed post. There was no window open or ceiling fan on. I feel it is Rocky's way to tell me he is okay.

It was not until after Christmas where I had a day where I wouldn't sit and cry for hours at a time. Molly was becoming more depressed and would not leave the front area hall of our home. I knew I needed to help her. Throughout this time, Ross had become my crutch. Ross helped me cope. His love, support, and patience over all of this brought us closer. Together, we knew we had to help Molly. I had to become stronger for the sake of her. Because Molly was used to having a friend around, the Vet suggested we think about getting another dog for her. The same friend, Johnny, who gave us Rocky, told us his daughter's dog had a litter and one of the pups needed a new home.

The girls knew Rocky was my dog. Molly seemed to be Lynn's dog. I promised Marie, the next dog would be hers. She was excited as we drove to see the pups. In the car Marie gave us suggestions on what its name would be. I suggested she sit on the floor and the dog that would belong to her would pick her.

Within seconds the chubbiest, black and white pup rolled over to her and squeaked. Marie gently picked him up and lovingly hugged him. Then he wet all over her t-shirt. Instantly, this pup had won over Marie's heart and picked his new owner. January 7th was the day he would come home with us. She named him, Willy.

In the meantime, we had to figure out how to help Molly. Her health was going down hill. I was very concerned about her. Ross suggested we let her play with his Jack Russell, Madie. Perhaps

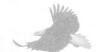

being around another dog, would pull Molly out of the depression. Molly and I walked over to the park and met Ross with Madie. At the same time, Marie was coming out of school and met Ross. Marie was deeply impressed at the effect Ross had on Molly. Molly, a dog we rescued from a shelter, who had been abused as a pup, didn't usually take to men at all, but she was all over Ross. Marie looked at this as a sign. Marie leaned into me and whispered, "This is the man I want you to marry, Mom." I was speechless. Marie is a very intuitive child. She certainly got me thinking. Ross was kind, gentle, with a wonderful loving heart. Most importantly to me, he was good with animals. He helped me through such a difficult time. He gave me unconditional love, a love that I had never had before except from Rocky. I decided it was time to tell the girls I was in love. Ross agreed.

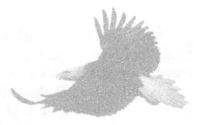

CHAPTER 33
Combining Families Is Not Easy

Can you do anything to change this situation?
If so, change it.
If not, let it go and stop worrying.
Let nature take its course.

Ross had also been married before. He had two girls of his own. They lived with their mother. Meeting his two girls was difficult. I wasn't sure how they would react, if they knew how serious we were about each other. I think they thought I was just another new girlfriend. Ross had dated five other women in the ten years since his divorce. I think they felt our relationship was a passing fling. Our two older girls knew each other from school. They were the same age. Because none of them knew how serious we were, they planned days when we wouldn't have them with us. His oldest, Kay, would make plans to go to a friend's, while Lynn would make plans for both my girls to go to their grandparents for a sleepover. The older girls secretly shared how it would be cool if we got married. Little did they know that we had been talking about marriage.

When Ross told his girls how much in love he was with me, his girls flipped. In the past the girls had Ross' complete attention and now he was sharing his attention with me and my two girls. Ross' youngest daughter, Beth, who was eleven at the time, wrote him a letter. In this letter she kept asking, "What about me Dad, what about me?" Her words and actions cried out for more attention. Kay was quiet and didn't say much. She was in shock. Lynn was very excited on the outside, but jealous and insecure on the inside. She wasn't sure where she would fit in. I think she was afraid she would lose me. Marie was thrilled. She had become very close to Ross. She said she felt like she was finally going to have a Dad who cared and truly loved her.

The varied reactions from the four girls, was a challenge for us. We didn't see it coming. Ross struggled regarding what to do about the choice Beth had given him. He was hurt by her words and selfish wishes. Ross sat Beth down and explained how for the first time in such a very long time he was completely happy and very much in love. Ross explained with tears in his eyes, "I want both of you in my life. My heart has plenty of love to share." He continued to explain, "As you get older, you will spend less and less time with me. Your friends and boys will fill your time. I don't want to grow old and be alone. I want to share my life with Sue." The more he talked about his loneliness in the past, and the love he had for me, the more she put walls up. That was the last conversation they shared. Her mother never encouraged her to see Ross ever again. In time, I know this child will come around, and perhaps even feel sad for all the happy times she missed with her father and us as a family. We all make choices in life and others have to respect that, and go on.

I promised my children, if I were ever to remarry, the man was going to have to ask them for permission. Unlike what happened when Robert got married, I wanted them included in the entire process. Ross took Lynn and Marie to Tim Horton's for a drink and donut and popped the question. Lynn screamed and made quite a scene in the restaurant. Ross later shared with me, how it was extremely embarrassing. When they got home Lynn came running into my room and spilled the beans. She told me he was about to propose. What she didn't know was Ross had already asked me a few days earlier. He didn't want to ask them and get them excited, and then I turned him down. I acted surprised when Lynn gave away the secret. From that moment on, we had problems with Lynn; she was mouthy and not following house rules. No homework was getting done, she was skipping school, and she was misbehaving all the time. A difficult side of her was appearing, one that I was never aware of before. It would be a good many years before things would work out for her. That is another book altogether.

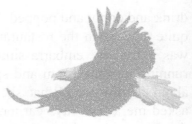

CHAPTER 34
My New Career

"We act as though comfort and luxury were the chief requirements of life, when all that we need to make us really happy is something to be enthusiastic about."

-Charles Kingsley

February 28, 2003 was the day my first children's book, "Rocky's Trip To The Hospital", was published. It felt like I had just given birth to a new baby. The feeling was like that of great accomplishment. I was proud. That day, when I held the finished book, I had no idea the positive impact it would have on many people. This book was written for children. To my pleasant surprise, half the purchases have been made for adults who use it as a tool to keep them positive in their life.

Within months, one of the major bookstores, Coles, had picked up my book and I was doing book signings up to five days per week. I was meeting lots of people who needed to hear my message. Because the book was about pet therapy, I brought Molly or Willy and we helped people heal through the healing power of pet therapy. It was very rewarding making that difference in people's lives.

Not too long after, another major bookstore, Chapters, got wind of what I was doing. They liked the effect my presence and the dogs were having on their customers. They picked up my book and we started book signings in their stores also.

It was at this time when I met another 'meant to be' person in my life, Judy Suke. While at a networking event one evening, this lovely lady came up to me during the break and said, "I can help you in your career." I was impressed and had a very strong, good feeling about her. Judy was also a member of Toastmasters. Interestingly enough we had never connected at any of their events. The time might not have been right, now I was ready for her.

Judy worked with me privately; preparing speeches with me, giving me tips on how to present myself, and showing me how to deliver my speeches in a confident, poised, and professional way. From the start she said that she believed in my message and knew that I could be a great speaker. I would not be where I am today, if it weren't for Judy coming into my life. This talented lady has a real gift for taking someone and helping them become powerful speakers.

The first speech we prepared together was, The Healing Power of Pets. This was basically me sharing my life story of what Rocky had done for me in my life. I delivered it for the first time in a Chapters bookstore followed by a book signing. As I gave that speech, the audience listened with great attention. Many of them had tears in their eyes, just like the group did at Toastmasters that first time when I delivered Rocky's story. After giving it, many people shared their experiences of pet therapy or asked questions regarding where the best place to adopt a pet would be, or how they could help more animals. It was more confirmation that I was doing the right thing in my life. I had touched many people just by sharing my story of healing with the help of Rocky. This was a great boost for my confidence.

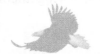

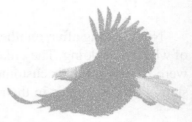

CHAPTER 35
Helping the Children Heal

"Reflect upon your present blessings, of which every man has plenty; not on your past misfortunes, of which all men have some."

-Charles Dickens

Seeing the affect the dogs had on people at my book signings, I wanted to take it a step further. I contacted our local children's hospital. I shared my story of being an author, and expressed my wish to come in and read my book to the children. I offered to do pet therapy and help them, just as Rocky had done for me when I was in the hospital. The staff loved the idea.

My first visit went great. Ross and Willy were at my side. With a group of sick children sitting around me, I introduced Willy as a friend of Rocky. I told them Rocky was a dog, that helped me heal, and Willy had come to help them feel better. I read the children my book, while Ross did pet therapy with the parents. After the children heard "Rocky's Trip To The Hospital", they felt strength and hope that their health would improve. They thought it was pretty cool to have an author come in and read to them, and give them autographs. While I was reading to the children, Ross shared our story about my health issues with the families, giving them hope for a brighter future. They felt I was a walking miracle. If it could happen for me, then it could happen for their children too.

On my next visit to the hospital, the staff shared positive things that had happened. Children had gone home sooner than expected. I had given them the mindset that they could get better. I was asked to visit with the children, who had more serious health issues. Children who were bedridden and could not come out to the lounge to hear the story or visit Willy. Unfortunately, Willy was not allowed to leave the lounge area and visit the wards. Although the children on the intensive care wards were often terminal, I decided that I could handle it. I told myself, "I must be ready for this, because it has come my way." The staff prepared me for what I would see, so I was not shocked to see a child that may perhaps be missing an arm or leg, or have all kinds of tubes hooked up to them.

After doing the usual reading in the lounge, with Willy and Ross doing their person to person pet therapy, I signed autographs, and gave out stickers that said, "I am a friend of Rocky." I told the children that, whenever they got scared of upcoming tests, surgeries, or were simply missing their normal life, they could put on this sticker, rub it, and know that Rocky was at their side. His spirit would give them strength and help them feel better and get through it. The sticker was another positive reminder that helped them heal and stay strong.

Going room to room, I read to the children, gave out stickers and coloring pages, and autographed pictures of me with the dogs. After my visit, some of the children I spoke to, even found strength to come to the lounge and visit the dog. This amazed the nurses and parents that these same children, who earlier were lying colorless, focusing on pain, and depressed; now, after spending time with me, wanted to see a dog. The children loved the idea that an author was giving them a ride in their wheelchair. We shared many laughs, and hugs. During these room visits, I gave the children tips on how I focused away from the pain. I shared how Rocky would lick my legs and breathe loudly into my ears. I taught them how to use visualization as a way to get away from their pain. Many of them visualized taking a trip to Disney World and meeting Mickey Mouse.

After the staff received more positive comments and saw what I was doing, I was then asked to visit children who were dying. I wasn't sure if I could handle it, however, I focused on the belief that this was coming to me for a reason. I knew I could help them, as I had experienced some of their feelings. I believed in my heart that the parents would hold on to my miracle healing story and that would help them cope.

The first child I visited was a cute, two-and-a-half-year old girl. She was small for her age and fragile-looking. She had Leukemia and was in the final stage. Before I entered the room, I asked God to give me strength to help this family cope. I could feel death in the room as I walked in. The little girl was crying, cuddled in her mother's arms. As I observed the scene, I was overwhelmed with sadness, and became intent on my effort to ease their pain. I put on a happy face, introduced myself, and offered to read my story to them.

The mother was grateful for some positive energy and seeing a new face. As I started to read, the little girl stopped crying, and began to smile. Her mother began to cry.

I thought, "What am I doing wrong here?" "Why is the mother crying?"

I guess the mother read the puzzled look on my face. She quickly explained, "My baby has not stopped crying for so long, and you have brought a smile to her tiny face. I thank you for being an angel in our life."

It was extremely challenging for me to keep it together. In that moment, I felt the power of my past experiences on my ability to help people. I knew that I was on a mission that was bigger than me. I also knew that I would be able to handle whatever God gave me to do. I autographed the book, gave it to them, and told the mother, "Keep this book as a memory of our time together."

I left the room and cried and cried. Ross brought me the dog to help me find some strength. I gathered my strength, pulled myself together and made a visit to four more rooms that morning. While walking out of the hospital, I said to Ross, "I have to put a book together that will give children strength when we can't be here." Ross assured me, "If anyone can do it, you can."

Later that night, at 3:00 a.m., I woke up with thoughts for my second book clearly in my mind. The title would be, "Rocky's Positive Thoughts Coloring Book". There would be pictures of children of all nationalities. The scenes would depict positive statements, such as, "Miracles do happen." "You were born to do great things." "Everything happens for a reason." Not wanting to wake up the household I took my notebook and went in to sit on the bathroom floor. Within half an hour the entire book was laid out. The actual scenes played in my mind.

One year later, on yet another visit to the hospital, I received heart-warming news. As I approached Ross, who had Willy in the lounge, I saw a familiar face. It was a boy I had visited months earlier. Jerome had been sitting anxiously with his father waiting to share some news with us. Jerome had just been informed that his cancer was in remission. He told us that the visualization techniques I had taught him, had helped him to heal, and by reading my books, he found the inner strength to cope and stay strong.

Both Ross and I gave him and his father a huge hug. I cried and Ross' eyes were a little wet also. That day was my birthday. I told Jerome, he had given me the nicest birthday present I could have ever received. He made me realize that I was truly living my life's

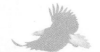

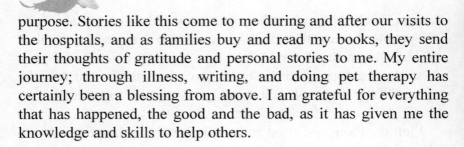

purpose. Stories like this come to me during and after our visits to the hospitals, and as families buy and read my books, they send their thoughts of gratitude and personal stories to me. My entire journey; through illness, writing, and doing pet therapy has certainly been a blessing from above. I am grateful for everything that has happened, the good and the bad, as it has given me the knowledge and skills to help others.

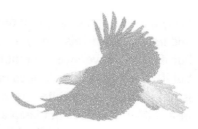

CHAPTER 36
The Beginning Of
Our New Life

"People are always blaming their circumstances for what they are. I do not believe in circumstances. The people who get on in this world are the people who get up and look for the circumstances they want, and if they cannot find them, make them."

-George Bernard Shaw

Ross and I got married November 29, 2003. The wedding was held in our home. Ross, his daughter Kay and our dog, Willy walked down the aisle together. My daughter Marie, and our other dog Molly, escorted me down the aisle. A small number of caring family and friends stood along the sides. It was a magical day. The house was filled with love. Our dear friend, Lloyd, delivered a touching reading at our ceremony with tremendous joy in his heart and a look that said "I told you so!" This is part of that reading: St. Paul's first letter to The Corinthians, Chapter 13: Verses 1-7 found in The New Testament of The Bible.

"I may be able to speak the languages of men and even angels, but if I don't have love, my speech is no more than a noisy gong or clanging bell.

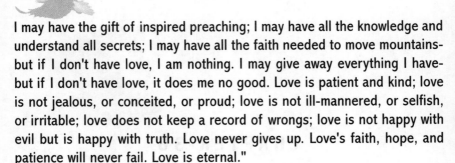
I may have the gift of inspired preaching; I may have all the knowledge and understand all secrets; I may have all the faith needed to move mountains- but if I don't have love, I am nothing. I may give away everything I have- but if I don't have love, it does me no good. Love is patient and kind; love is not jealous, or conceited, or proud; love is not ill-mannered, or selfish, or irritable; love does not keep a record of wrongs; love is not happy with evil but is happy with truth. Love never gives up. Love's faith, hope, and patience will never fail. Love is eternal."

For our honeymoon we went to Hawaii for three amazing weeks. We had wanted to go first class, yet did not want to spend the extra money. The universe responded, and as a surprise wedding gift to us, Ross' sister and brother-in-law gave us an envelope with executive class plane tickets.

This trip was a dream come true! I had been longing to go to Hawaii for 25 years. I had visualized the beaches, the flowers and the beautiful blue ocean. It was a very long trip. The flight was a total of 14 hours with switching planes in different airports. When we landed on that Maui runway at 11 p.m., I had tears running down my cheeks. It was a moment of extreme pride. I had accomplished so much. I was extremely grateful. I was grateful to have my health, to be able to make this trip with confidence and without fear. I was grateful for the people who had played such an important part in my healing process. I was thrilled to have someone to love and share the experience with.

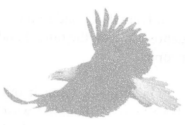

CHAPTER 37
Soaring

"If you are walking in the right direction, all you need to do is keep on walking."

-Buddist Proverb

Our Deepest Fear

"Our deepest fear is not that we are inadequate. Our deepest fear is that we are powerful beyond measure. It is our light, not our darkness, that most frightens us. We ask ourselves, 'Who am I to be brilliant, gorgeous, talented and fabulous?' Actually, who are you not to be? You are a child of God. Your playing small doesn't serve the world. There's nothing enlightened about shrinking so that other people won't feel insecure around you. We were born to make manifest the glory of God that is within us. It's not just in some of us; it's in everyone. And as we let our light shine, we unconsciously give other people the permission to do the same. As we are liberated from our own fear, our presence automatically liberates others."

- Nelson Mandela, 1994 Inaugural Speech

I knew that until I faced every fear in my life, I would not be able to completely soar and become successful. I still had some

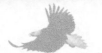

final fears that I had to face. On the one hand, I was terrified of the dentist; and on the other hand I feared being around successful, rich people.

Once again, I put it out there, that my intention was to face these fears. Although, I wasn't sure how it would happen, I knew if I asked I would receive the help I needed.

The fear of going to the dentist had haunted me all my life. Weeks before every visit I would begin to feel nauseous, I couldn't sleep, and I would begin to panic. The night before the appointment, I would spend hours in the washroom with diarrhea and vomiting. The memory of what happened when I got my wisdom teeth removed was buried deep within my cells. I had to deal with this fear in order to go forward. I had dealt with a lot in my life and had overcome many challenges. The time had come to get over this fear. I knew I needed help with it.

Just days after making this decision, a situation led me to my answer. I was at Marie's swimming lessons in our local YMCA. I felt compelled to go over to the counter and read a pamphlet. After glancing quickly at it, I told the girl at the counter I had to book a treatment with a healer named Linda Powell. Linda did various alternative health treatments. One of those treatments was called Integrated Energy Therapy. The focus of this therapy is to clear suppressed cellular memories and emotions that create blockages. It works on physical, emotional, mental and spiritual levels; clearing the blockages and helping a person to discover their soul's mission in life. Integrated Energy Therapy clears energy blocks that limit your health, life purpose, prosperity and creativity. Linda, through her therapy, helped me to reach my full potential.

Not long after the first treatment with Linda, a thought came to me. Rocky had helped me cope with many situations, why not have my dog, Molly help me through the fear of the dentist? I contacted my dentist and told him I had an idea. He said, "Sue, I am willing to try anything with you at this point." Dr. Handa knew of the experiences I had with pet therapy. I actually chose him as my dentist, because he had a fish tank in his waiting room. Fish have been proven to calm people. The night before going for a couple of fillings, I found myself to be calmer than I had been in the past. I felt courageous just knowing that Molly would be there by my side. I knew if Dr. Handa did anything bad to me, Molly would take a chunk out of him. (Not really, but the thought was comforting.)

Ross came with me to the dentist appointment. Not only was he there to support me, he could take care of Molly if something went wrong. We had never taken a dog to the dentist and I wasn't sure how she would react to the sound of the drill. We were all surprised by how much the dog helped me.

I got into the chair, and as if on cue, Molly sprawled her body over mine; laying her head on my chest and putting her paws around my neck as if to comfort me. She sat the entire time just looking into my eyes. I focused deeply into her big brown eyes, while I rubbed her furry soft ears. Once again my pet had come to the rescue to help me cope with a challenging situation. Linda's treatment brought me the solution.

When I began writing this book, I had to stop after a week, due to having such tremendous pain in my stomach. Because my cells had stored all the negative and painful memories of what I had been through, I started reliving my life with each word I wrote. I started having flashbacks and nightmares. I was amazed at how, although I was physically better, I hadn't healed emotionally and this too was holding me back. I didn't think I would ever complete this book. After another treatment with Linda, she cleared the cells of the negative memories and this allowed me to write from my heart. I sat down and wrote for hours after each treatment. The words poured out of me. The memories were only that, memories. I had no pain or feeling associated with it any longer.

Growing up, I had the belief that people who had money were either, snobbish or bad, or both. Why would I want to be like them? Therefore I had not created a desire to be rich. Also, statements from people in my past had convinced me that I did not deserve to be rich. I didn't fully value myself or my work and because of that I did not ask for adequate pay. These were only my 'beliefs', and were holding me back from reaching my full potential.

My next treatment I wanted to clear my thoughts around success and money. Once again the treatment did the trick. During the session, I got a clear vision of my future. In one scene, I saw myself on stage, a young granddaughter, about age three or four was holding my hand, while I was speaking in front of 5,000 people. In other scenes, I saw all the books I would write and the people I would help. I saw the difference Ross, our children and I were making in our world. I saw the homes we would have. While I was out speaking and doing book signings, Ross was holding down the fort on a ranch. One of our future goals is to have our own ranch and do pet therapy with disabled children and horses. That was clearly established in my vision.

One of my past problems was I didn't believe where my life was heading. By seeing this vision, I started to truly believe, and in fact, know it is part of my mission in life, to be successful and have money to help others. I have come to realize that you need to create a clear vision of your 'perfect' life, in order to recognize the opportunities that come your way. When you do this, the universe will bring you what you need; the people, the things, and the experiences to create your reality.

Not long after this treatment, I received a phone call from a wonderful friend, Karen Zizzo. She said she wanted to share a business opportunity with Ross and me. Because we accept that things happen for a reason, we were completely open to learning about this opportunity. During our meeting with Karen, both Ross and I knew we had to become involved with this business. The business is called, InterBIZ. It is an internet business that saves people time and money and develops a passive residual income. It would also help me with time management by delivering my products to my door. No longer did I have to run errands and waste time in long lines. We would have the opportunity to improve our business skills. This business held every benefit we were looking for. Plus, it gave us another opportunity to be able to help more people in the future.

Once again there was a much bigger plan for us getting involved with this business. New doors continuously open each day. We are meeting a lot of terrific new people who are kind, supportive, and spiritual. Ross and I are able to help people become financially free, and grow as individuals. We are bringing hope back to many people. Karen has become like the big sister I never had. We help each other reach our goals by being accountable to each other.

As the business grows for us, Ross and I see the potential for Ross getting the opportunity to retire from his full-time job. For months, we had discussed our options on how I could be in two places at once. I didn't want to go on a speaking or book tour until Ross could be home with Marie. I refused to accept her coming home to a lonely house while I was out having a career. After coming to this decision, we met with someone else in the business, Rod Schulhauser. He was an engineer who retired due to this business. Once again, when the student is ready, the teacher will appear. Rod became our mentor and coach. Whenever you want to reach a goal, having a mentor or coach is one of the best ways to do it. Look for someone who has already become successful. Pick someone who is walking his talk. Rod has mentored us and kept us on track for reaching our goals. When he has seen it is time for us to kick it up a level and do something new, he let's us know. We don't let him down.

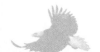

When we got comfortable with being around our mentor, Rod, we met someone at a higher level in the business. We have been blessed and fortunate to meet the founder of InterBIZ, Casey Combden. This was the final piece of my puzzle that had to be solved in order for me to soar.

Remember my opinion of people with money; that they are snobbish or bad. Because of this belief, I was terrified of being around anyone with lots of money. When I first met Casey I was shaking and couldn't make eye contact with him. I felt he was judging me and I felt inferior to him. It was all in my head! I knew I had to get over this if I was going to become successful. Once again, another treatment with Linda helped me.

I no longer avoided being around the leaders in the business. In fact, I actively went out of my way to participate in their events. I knew if I was around Casey I would see the real him. He is a man who is kind, generous, and extremely spiritual.

It didn't take long for him to know who I was. After one of our encounters he commented to Rod, "She's going to make it!" Casey, being intuitive, had a sense about me. It was a positive feeling and more confirmation that I was on track. The more time I was around Casey, the more I saw him as just a regular guy. He was a person, who just like me, wanted to make a positive difference for many people in our world. He was spiritual, not snobby. He was a good person, not bad. While having dinner one evening with Casey and his wife, Jeannie, and other business people, I asked Casey what he felt I needed to work on in my life to grow to the next level. He looked at me, smiled, and said, "You have faced all your fears, you have conquered your challenges from the past, now you will only be successful." That was the biggest confirmation I have ever received in my life.

I was ready to soar!

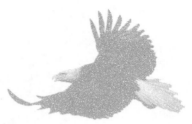

My Final Thoughts

I have had many challenges to conquer, many fears to face, and in order to soar, had to become my own person. When the time is right, when you have faced your challenges, you too will be ready to soar. In the meantime, enjoy life and live in the now! Be grateful for every gift that God sends your way. There are no endings, only new beginnings. Have complete trust that God will provide all that you need in your life.

I wish you love, laughter, and happiness!
All the best,
Love Sue

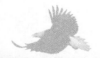

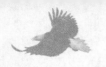

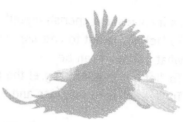

Quotes and Poems
to Help You Soar

LET GO

To "let go" does not mean to stop caring, it means I can't do it for someone else

To "let go" is not to cut myself off, it's the realization I can't control another person

To "let go" is not to enable, but to allow learning from natural consequences

To "let go" is to admit powerlessness, which means the outcome is not in my hands

To "let go" is not to try to change or blame another, it's to make the most of myself

To "let go" is not to care for, but to care about

To "let go" is not to fix, but to be supportive

To "let go" is not to judge, but to allow another to be a human being, flaws and all

To "let go" is not to be in the middle arranging all the out comings but to allow others to affect their own destinies

To "let go" is not to be protective, it's to permit another to face reality

To "let go" is not to deny, but to accept

To "let go" is not to nag, scold or argue, but instead to search out my own shortcomings and correct them

To "let go" is not to adjust everything to my desires but to take each day

as it comes and cherish myself in it
To "let go" is not to criticize and regulate anybody but to try to become what I dream I can be
To "let go" is not to regret the past, but to grow and live for the future
To "let go" is to fear less and love more

Poem from The Association of Parent Support Groups in Ontario newsletter

IF DOGS COULD TEACH

If a dog was the teacher, you would learn stuff like....

When loved ones come home, always run to greet them.

Never pass up the opportunity to go for a joyous ride.

Allow the experience of fresh air and the wind in your face to be pure ecstasy.

When it's in your best interest, practice obedience.

Let others know when they've invaded your territory.

Take naps.

Stretch before rising.

Run, romp, and play daily.

Thrive on attention and let people touch you.

Avoid biting when a simple growl will do.

On warm days, stop to lie on your back on the grass.

On hot days, drink lots of water and lie under a shady tree.

When you're happy, dance around and wag your entire body.

No matter how often you're scolded, don't buy into the guilt thing and pout...run right back and make friends.

Delight in the simple joy of a long walk.

Eat with gusto and enthusiasm. Stop when you have had enough.

Be loyal. Never pretend to be something you are not.

If what you want lies buried, dig until you find it.

When someone is having a bad day, be silent, sit close by and nuzzle them gently.

-Author Unknown

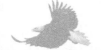

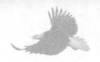

<u>Parent's Proverbs</u>

Your resources are limited
-Emotional and Financial

If you continue to blame yourself,
You will continue to be helpless;

Your child's behavior affects how you behave,
Your behavior affects how your child will behave;

Children have responsibilities as well as rights,
Parents have rights as well as responsibilities;

Harmony and co-operation can replace
Anarchy and confusion;

Taking a stand can cause a crisis,
When you take the stand,
You can control the crisis;

Positive change will result
when you respond thoughtfully.

-The Association of Parent Support Groups in Ontario

<u>Dreams Are.......</u>

Dreams are a big part of our lives
And you must do whatever it takes
To make them a reality;
By the plans you make,
The course you take,
And the things you do.

Don't dwell on past mistakes.
Leave yesterday behind,
Along with all its problems,
worries and doubts.

Realize you can't change the past,
But you can start a new tomorrow.
Don't try to do everything at once;
Take one step at a time,

Don't ever be afraid to try the impossible
No matter what others may think.
Remember you are unique
In your own special way.

Don't ever stop Dreaming!
Don't ever stop wanting what's right for you!

-an e-card sent to me from Ross

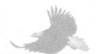

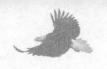

Things To Do Each Day

Tear this page out and stick on your refrigerator

Appreciate your uniqueness.
Assess your talents.
Take the necessary steps.
Know you can do it.
Keep your dreams alive.
Overcome obstacles.
Let your spirit soar.
Reach out.
Think big.
Rejoice in your capabilities.
Take a giant leap forward.
Believe in yourself.
Hold tightly to dreams.
Never give up.
Ask for help.
Be patient.
See opportunity everywhere.
Live each day.
Open your heart.
Expect the best.
Love for the sake of loving.

Build on your strengths.
Make a fresh start.
Envision success.
Imagine the possibilities.
Savor your strength.
Stay happy.
Launch new ideas.
Aim high.
Live fully.
Invest in your potential.
Don't look back.
Seize the moment.
Never lose hope
Be alive.
Have the courage to change.
Keep promises.
Love each moment.
Build a better tomorrow.
Explore your soul.
Let miracles happen.
Give for the sake of giving

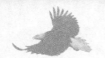

Sample Affirmations Created By Sue London

(By repeating positive phrases and feeling inside as if they are here, you can create a new reality)

Affirmations to Confirm Wealth

I am prosperous.

I see abundance all around me and my life is blessed.

I attract success on every level.

I am learning to attract more opportunities to make money.

Affirmations to Confirm Health

I enjoy physical exercise and working out is a pleasure.

I plan ahead and always have time to exercise.

I have a body that radiates health and energy.

Water is healthy for my body. I cleanse my body with 8 glasses of water per day.

I eat lots for fresh fruits and vegetables.

I always stop eating when I have had enough.

I eat three balanced meals per day.

I limit my sugar intake.

Mind and body is one thing and I listen to the nutritional needs of my body.

I eat plenty of natural food with high fibre content.

Affirmations to Confirm Strength and Courage

I am a lucky man/woman/child.

I focus on the positive and many good things effortlessly come my way.

I soar towards excellence.

I am balanced and content.

I naturally attract winners into my life.

I deserve to be loved, honored, and respected.

I overcome adversity and create new beginnings.

My house reflects my inner being and I enjoy keeping it clean.

I recognize signs of disrespect towards me and my children and act appropriately.

I conquer my fears of the future by surrounding myself with positive people.

I build my confidence by learning new skills.

171

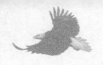

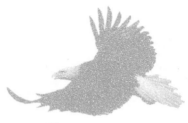

Other Books by Sue London

Rocky's Journey
Children's book series that help children heal from life's most challenging situations

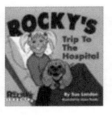

Rocky's Trip To The Hospital
(ISBN 0-9732158-0-1)

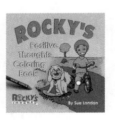

Rocky's Positive Thoughts Coloring Book
(ISBN 0-9732158-1-X)

For more information about contacting Sue London as a speaker and Life & Success Coach, visit her web site at www.rockysjourney.com

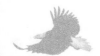

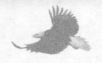

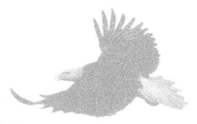

Recommended Reading

Albom, Mitch, Tuesdays with Morrie, New York: Random House, 1997

Andrews, Ted, Animal- Speak, St. Paul, Mn: Llewellyn Publications, 2000

Ball, Pamela, 10,000 Dreams Interpreted, Great Britain: Arcturus Publishing, 1996

Becker, Marty Dr., The Healing Powers of Pets, New York: Hyperion, 2002

Bristol, Claude M., The Magic of Believing, New York: Fireside, 1991

Canfield, Jack, The Success Principles: How to Get from Where You Are to Where You Want to Be, New York: Harper Collins, 2005

Carson, Richard Dr., Don't Sweat The Small Stuff About Money, New York: Hyperion, 2001

Dyer, Wayne W. Dr, Manifest Your Destiny, New York: Harper Collins, 1997

Dyer, Wayne W. Dr., The Power of Intention, Carlsbad, California: Hay House Inc, 2004

Hay, Louise L., You Can Heal Your Life, Carlsbad, California: Hay House Inc, 1984

Pretorius, Elfreda, Rules of the Game- How to Overcome struggle. Victoria, Canada: Trafford, 2004

Redfield, James, The Celestine Prophecy, New York: Warner Books, 1993

Sharma, Robin S., The Monk Who Sold His Ferrari, Toronto, Canada: Harper Collins, 1997

Siegel, Bernie S. M.D., Peace, Love & Healing, New York: Harper Collins, 1989

Spiller, Jan, Astrology For The Soul, New York: Bantam Books, 1997

Vincent Zizzo, Karen. Ask and You Shall Receive- A Miracle for Steven. Ancaster, Canada: Enlightening Publishing, 2004

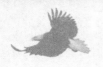